Language Treatment and Generalization

Language Treatment and Generalization

A Clinician's Handbook

Diana L. Hughes, PhD
Department of Communication Disorders
Central Michigan University

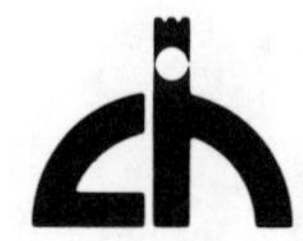

COLLEGE-HILL PRESS, San Diego, California

College-Hill Press, Inc.
4284 41st Street
San Diego, California 92105

Library of Congress Cataloging in Publication Data
Main entry under title:

Hughes, Diana L., 1947-
Language treatment and generalization.

Bibliography: p.
Includes index.
1. Language disorders—Treatment. I. Title.
RC423.H83 1985 616.85′5 85-5750

ISBN 0-88744-145-9

Printed in the United States of America

CONTENTS

PREFACE

This book was begun as the result of encouragement from a colleague, Giri Hegde, with whom the author presented a miniseminar at the 1983 American Speech-Language-Hearing Association convention in Cincinnati. The miniseminar, titled "Language Training and Generalization: The Clinician's Dilemma," was well-attended, and many requests for copies of the handouts were received. There seemed to be a receptive audience of practicing clinicians for whom the "dilemma" was quite real. Furthermore, a search of available literature revealed no convenient source of information on generalization that was specifically tailored to the language intervention process.

As the book began to take shape, working clinicians were the reading audience kept firmly in mind. For that reason, the summaries of scientific research included in this book are somewhat detailed, often including some description of the subjects and specific details about procedures and measures. The summaries were written to be thorough enough for clinicians to try out some ideas from the research literature after reading this book. Discussion of research results and conclusions concerning generalization strategies are data-based and presented in a pragmatic style designed to encourage application of strategies and questions for future research.

Many of the experimental studies described in this book used single-subject research designs and came from behaviorally oriented journals. Under the assumption that the research background of many clinicians probably emphasized only large group research, a brief section describing multiple-baseline and reversal or withdrawal designs is included in Chapter 2. For readers who have not been exposed to within-subject research designs, this brief introduction should prove beneficial. Perhaps clinicians will be encouraged to try some clinical research of their own.

Thus, one of the possible outcomes of this book is an increase in clinical research investigating the various factors thought to influence generalization effects of language treatment. Clinician-readers may find themselves considering their caseloads for potential subjects with whom to try a generalization tactic. There is a great need for well-controlled clinical research, and the various within-subject designs are well-suited to the practicing clinician who has lots of questions but few answers.

Readers will note the prevalence of behaviorist-oriented language intervention research described in the following chapters. This is a result not so much of any bias on the part of the author, but of the kinds of published research that have specifically investigated the phenomena of generalization. In searching the literature pertaining to generalization of language subsequent to therapy or treatment, many of the relevant studies were found in behaviorally oriented journals. Indeed, the term *generalization* itself is closely associated with behaviorist theory. There are psycholinguistically oriented studies of language intervention, but these rarely include specific measures of generalization, in addition to acquisition, of language behaviors or skills.

This book is not meant to be explanatory—many questions concerning generalization remain unanswered. No doubt if more were understood about it, our clinical language intervention would be more successful. However, it does not follow that, lacking such understanding, our work is doomed to failure. As Crystal (1983) so aptly phrased it, "... It is commonplace to achieve success, without knowing how we did it" (p. 6).

Several persons contributed to the growth of my interest in, and understanding of, the process of generalization as part of language intervention. Notable among these were my four dissertation subjects, Mark, Michael, Marita, and Ryan. I am especially indebted to my colleague Giri Hegde, who by correspondence and direct discussion has added to my understanding of the complexities of generalization and maintenance issues in language treatment. I am grateful for his comments and feedback on most of the chapters in the book. I am also grateful to Monica McHenry for her comments on early drafts of each chapter and to Carl Johnson for his comments on the chapter on maintenance and the section on within-subject designs.

Preparation of this manuscript was made possible by a Summer Research Fellowship from Central Michigan University, for which I am very grateful. I also wish to thank all of my friends and colleagues whose support contributed to this effort.

D.L.H.
Mt. Pleasant, Michigan

Chapter 1

Definitions of Generalization

THE OTHER HALF OF THE JOB—WHY GENERALIZATION IS IMPORTANT

Speech-language clinicians who work with language-disordered clients strive to establish improved language skills or behaviors. Experimental clinical literature has shown that improvement is possible, at least when measured within the treatment setting (Costello, 1983; Leonard, 1981; Rogers-Warren and Warren, 1981). However, generalization of such learned skills to nontreatment environments, such as school classrooms, home, work environments, and play environments, often fails to occur. Unless some degree of generalization occurs across settings, people, times, and visual and verbal stimuli other than those used in treatment, clinicians should seriously question the impact of their language intervention programs.

Establishing a desired language behavior within a limited environment is a necessary first step toward successful language intervention. But clients rarely confine their language use to such limited environments. Since language behavior must be available for use in diverse situations, it is necessary first to *check* for generalization of the target behaviors, and if the degree of generalization is unsatisfactory, intervention must continue until an appropriate level of generalization is achieved.

Clinicians should not feel alone in facing the problem of generalization of behaviors taught in direct treatment. A large body of literature in psychology and education has described, explained, and attempted to remedy the problem of generalization failure (Kazdin, 1980; Marholin and Siegel, 1978; Marholin, Siegel, and Phillips, 1976; Wahler, Berland, and Coe, 1979). In 1977 a classic article by Stokes and Baer reviewed many experimental-behavioral studies, seeking common principles involved in successful generalization. As a result of reviewing some 120 studies in the generalization literature, Stokes and Baer derived nine general categories of techniques or methods used to examine, assess, or program generalization. One category consisted of studies that employed no specific programming to achieve generalization—the "train-

and-hope'' studies. Another category included studies in which generalization across several nontreatment conditions was assessed. If generalization was absent or deficient, systematic, sequential modifications were made to achieve it across each condition. The seven remaining categories constitute a core of generalization tactics, which were offered as a set of ''what-to-do'' possibilities and to spur future research. These tactics are summarized in Table 1–1. Keep in mind as you read them that these tactics are not specific to language behaviors. However, many of the studies described in subsequent chapters have employed some of these tactics or variations of them.

Since this earlier article, Baer (1981) has written a small booklet aimed toward anyone who is trying to bring about deliberate behavior changes in self or others, which summarizes ten steps to encourage generalization of behavior changes. Many of these steps are rewordings or combinations of those presented in Table 1–1.

GENERALIZATION DEFINED

For purposes of this book, the term generalization will be used rather broadly. A review of the generalization literature indicates that a variety of terms that appear to have interchangeable meanings have been used to describe similar phenomena, among them *generalization, transfer, carry-over, induction,* and *spread-of-effect*. While these terms may distinguish among various subtle differences within the broad concept, the generic term *generalization* has come to be used most commonly to describe the extension of some learning to new instances.

Normal Versus Disordered Language Learning

Generalization has been used to refer to many kinds of similar learning phenomena in both normal and disordered populations. It has been used to describe both language phenomena learned without direct teaching, as is the case with normal children, and phenomena that result from direct language teaching, as is the case with language-disordered children. From the literature on normal language development, clinicians are familiar with the notions of ''overgeneralization'' or ''overregularization'' of irregular verbs and plurals (e.g., *goed, mans*), which are typically observed in the course of normal language acquisition. These examples, in which a general rule is applied to irregular forms, may provide a good, albeit limited, beginning point for understanding the phenomena of generalization of language behavior. Within the normal

Table 1–1. Stokes and Baer's Generalization Tactics

1. Introduce the target behaviors to natural maintaining contingencies that will refine and maintain them without further intervention. Teach subjects to cue potential natural communities to reinforce desired behaviors.
2. Train sufficient exemplars; use enough different teachers, settings, and stimuli so that generalization across these parameters will occur. Diversify the exemplars.
3. Train loosely, using relatively little control over stimulus conditions or responses, so that variations occur. Train different examples concurrently and vary instructions and reinforcements.
4. Use indiscriminable contingencies; make the contingencies and setting events that mark them less predictable. Conceal the point at which contingencies stop operating.
5. Program common stimuli by including within treatment the social and physical stimuli that are salient and functional in natural environments. For example, use peer tutors.
6. Use mediated generalization; teach subjects to accurately self-record, self-reinforce, and self-report the target behaviors.
7. Train to generalize; reinforce generalization as if it were an operant response class.

learning literature, generalization is often synonymous with concept formation or rule learning.

Within the literature on language disorders and language intervention, the term *generalization* has been defined not from the perspective of a naturally occurring phenomenon during normal language development, but from a *treatment* perspective. When the phenomenon of language generalization is viewed from a treatment perspective, it differs from naturally occurring language generalization in two major ways. First, since treatment requires a deliberate attempt to *teach* some aspect of language, there are often specific antecedent events, such as verbal instructions or visual stimuli, which set up an opportunity to provide a specific language response. Although similar antecedent events may occur naturally, they are not deliberate or planned, but occur unsystematically and perhaps with low frequency.

The treatment perspective on generalization differs from the natural perspective in another way: the consequent events that follow a language behavior or an opportunity to produce a language behavior. During treatment, deliberate attempts are made to increase correct responding by systematically providing known (or assumed) positive reinforcers immediately after correct responses, or by providing punishment or no positive reinforcers after incorrect responses, or both. By contrast, both correct and incorrect language behaviors may be consequated quite unsystematically in the course of normal language learning. Sometimes children receive what may be assumed to be positive reinforcement for *incorrect* language, for example, the granting of a request after production of an ungrammatical and somewhat rude request, such as "Me want big piece." Likewise, children may *not* receive positive reinforcement for a grammatically correct polite request such as "May I please have a cookie, Mother?"; for example, this request may be denied. It may be assumed, however, from a behavioral perspective that grammatically correct and appropriate language is gradually shaped via some kind of positive reinforcement.

Both of these major differences between normal language learning and disordered language learning are crucial to the issue of language generalization. When clinical researchers define generalization, they must address the distinction between the kinds of naturally occurring antecedent events for language production and those that are deliberately programmed in the course of treatment. Likewise, clinical researchers must also consider the reinforcement that may be received as "natural reinforcement" in nontreatment environments and the often artificial reinforcers used in treatment.

A Definition of Generalization—and Some Problems

A frequently cited definition of generalization within an applied behavioral framework may provide a starting point for a discussion of generalization of language treatment effects. According to Stokes and Baer (1977), generalization may be defined as

> ... the occurrence of relevant behavior under different, nontraining conditions (i.e., across subjects, settings, people, behaviors, and/or time) without the scheduling of the same events in those conditions as had been scheduled in the training conditions. Thus, generalization may be claimed when no extratraining manipulations are needed for extratraining change; or may be claimed when some extra manipulations are necessary, but their cost or extent is clearly less than that of the direct intervention. Generalization will not be claimed when similar events are necessary for similar effects across conditions. (p. 350)

Several problems arise as this definition of generalization is considered. One problem concerns whether to distinguish between generalization that occurs without further intervention (i.e., "spontaneously") and generalization that is achieved after additional, "indirect" intervention. If the intervention effort is broken down into an *establishment* or training phase of the program, which can be distinguished from a *generalization* phase during which no direct "training" may occur, then what should any "extratraining manipulations" be called? Is this to be considered a new phase of the treatment program, one that is less direct and costly?

The "extratraining manipulations" part of the definition also raises questions. What constitutes manipulations that are clearly less in cost or extent than direct intervention?

The Stokes and Baer definition distinguishes between training and extratraining conditions. In addition to these two ways that generalization may occur, it is possible to conceive of a third version of the intervention effort, i.e., a treatment program that has been carefully designed from the start to promote generalization, rather than simply to establish target responses. If certain tactics are employed early in the intervention effort, generalization may occur "spontaneously" without the need for a generalization phase. Indeed, the major purpose of this book is to help clinicians begin to plan intervention in this way.

It might be useful, then, to distinguish among three different ways that generalization effects of language treatment may occur. These categories are shown in Table 1–2. The term *unplanned generalization* may be applied to the first category to describe generalization that occurs "spontaneously," after a period of traditional establishment-phase treatment. Without any additional programming, the language target is observed during some kind of generalization measure, for example, within spontaneous language samples in the child's home. Consider how many mildly language-delayed children have probably been released from treatment without a rigorous assessment of generalization. If they never appear on therapy caseloads again, it is likely to be because their language appears normal to parents or subsequent screeners. In these cases, maturation over time probably resulted in generalized use of trained language, or perhaps complete generalization and maintenance occurred immediately after training.

For the second category a special generalization phase of treatment is begun after results of a generalization measure indicate that the language target has not generalized to the desired conditions, or a very low rate or frequency of occurrence is observed. This may be called *post-hoc programmed generalization*.

The third category, *pre-planned generalization*, describes language intervention for which the entire treatment program is designed to facili-

Table 1–2. Ways to Distinguish Generalization of Language Behaviors Subsequent to Treatment

Category	Examples	Generalization occurred across:
1. No generalization program required. Generalization occurs "spontaneously" without direct effort to achieve it.	Clinician trains client to produce *he* and *she* correctly as subject pronouns in structured therapy tasks. At a later time, spontaneous language samples collected by parents at home show 100% correct production in at least 10 obligatory contexts for each pronoun.	Setting, persons, some response generalization across untrained sentence contexts; generalization to spontaneous production.
2. Generalization phase of treatment required. Generalization does not occur "spontaneously" but does occur with additional programming designed to achieve generalization across necessary parameters.	Clinician trains client to produce three-word Agent-Action-Object utterances in answer to "What-doing" questions and doll manipulations in structured therapy tasks. Within the classroom, the client does not respond or responds with one or two words to teacher questions and manipulations of a new doll. Subsequently, the teacher implements a generalization program designed to elicit three-word utterances in answer to questions.	Setting, person, different visual stimuli, possibly across untrained word combinations.
3. Generalization techniques built in to treatment program. Generalization occurs across several parameters because specific strategies to encourage such generalization are integrated into the initial treatment program.	Clinician and two other teachers train client to respond correctly to locative commands (e.g., "Put the penny under the box") in multiple settings with multiple objects and locations. Subsequently, parents report client telling siblings at home to place objects in various locations.	Setting, persons, modalities (receptive to expressive language), some response generalization across untrained examples; generalization to spontaneous production.

tate generalization across several parameters right from the start. As more is learned about how generalization is accomplished, these kinds of language intervention programs should become more common. Given the individual variation among clients, it is probable that all three categories of generalization will be observed.

A second problem in defining generalization, one that was not addressed by the Stokes and Baer definition, is the degree of consistency in performance required of the language target behavior under the generalization conditions in order to say that the behavior has generalized. For some language target behaviors there are many optional situations in which the behavior *may* occur but is not obligatory. The decision regarding when the behavior can be said to have generalized depends on what is viewed as an "appropriate" rate of occurrence in nontreatment environments. It may be impossible to determine a percentage of correct occurrence.

For other language target behaviors, e.g., grammatical targets, it is possible to determine where obligatory contexts occur and thus compute a percentage of correct occurrence. For determining that a particular grammatical morpheme was "acquired," Brown (1973) used the criterion of 90 per cent occurrence in obligatory contexts, and this standard has also been used in determining whether to include a particular morpheme as a therapy target (Tyack and Gottsleben, 1974). Hence, our goal in treating grammar deficits has been to achieve correct production in 90 per cent of the obligatory contexts that occur within a spontaneous language sample.

As the previous discussion has shown, the issues that are raised in trying to refine the concept of generalization as it relates to language intervention are many. In an attempt to bring some structure and organization to a description of generalization, it may be useful at this point to break generalization down into subtypes along the lines used by behavioral-learning psychologists. Generalization is typically broken down into *stimulus generalization*, which can be further examined in terms of various stimulus parameters, and *response generalization*. In addition, generalization in its broader sense may also include generalization over time, or *maintenance*.

STIMULUS GENERALIZATION

There are many characteristics or parameters that differ between treatment and nontreatment conditions. Numerous aspects of the stimulus complex found in language treatment may be different from stimuli that can appropriately trigger language in nontreatment environments. Among the aspects that may vary between treatment and generalization conditions are the stimuli (e.g., the visual and verbal antecedents), persons, settings, and time. Figure 1–1 illustrates a number of these parameters that may vary between treatment and nontreatment environments.

Generalization may or may not occur in the presence of nontraining visual stimulus materials—and these could be as slightly different from the training stimuli as two different balls, a drawing of a ball versus a photograph of a ball, or even the same ball at a later time (perhaps scuffed and dirty). For some severely language-disordered children, successful generalization of a verbal label (e.g., *ball*), either receptively or expressively, across different examples of the referent may be a major accomplishment.

Generalization may also occur or fail to occur in the presence of nontraining verbal antecedents, e.g., "What's this?", "What is that?", or "Tell me the name of this thing." When the language target behavior is a more sophisticated language response, e.g., a grammatically correct coordinated sentence uttered appropriately within a conversation, the variety of nontraining verbal antecedents is probably infinite.

Generalization effects of language training can also be observed as the client talks to different people, using specific trained sentences or untrained generalized responses. The new listeners may come into the therapy room, or a language sample with a nontraining listener may be collected in a classroom or at home. In addition, new listeners may be found in groups, in contrast to the one-to-one clinician-client interaction that is typical in much direct language treatment. Generalization from one-to-many and from many-to-one may occur or fail to occur.

The learned language target may or may not generalize to different physical settings. Setting generalization may include moving physical objects in the training room to new locations within the room or moving therapy activities from floor to table. Often clinicians may arrange for therapy sessions to occur in nontraining locations such as university unions, outside the clinic or school, or in work locations. Clinicians may recall therapy sessions from their clinical practica that included visits to a snack bar or collection of language samples while sitting outside on the grass.

Response Generalization

In addition to stimulus generalization, a learned language target may also be said to generalize across responses or behaviors. In this case,

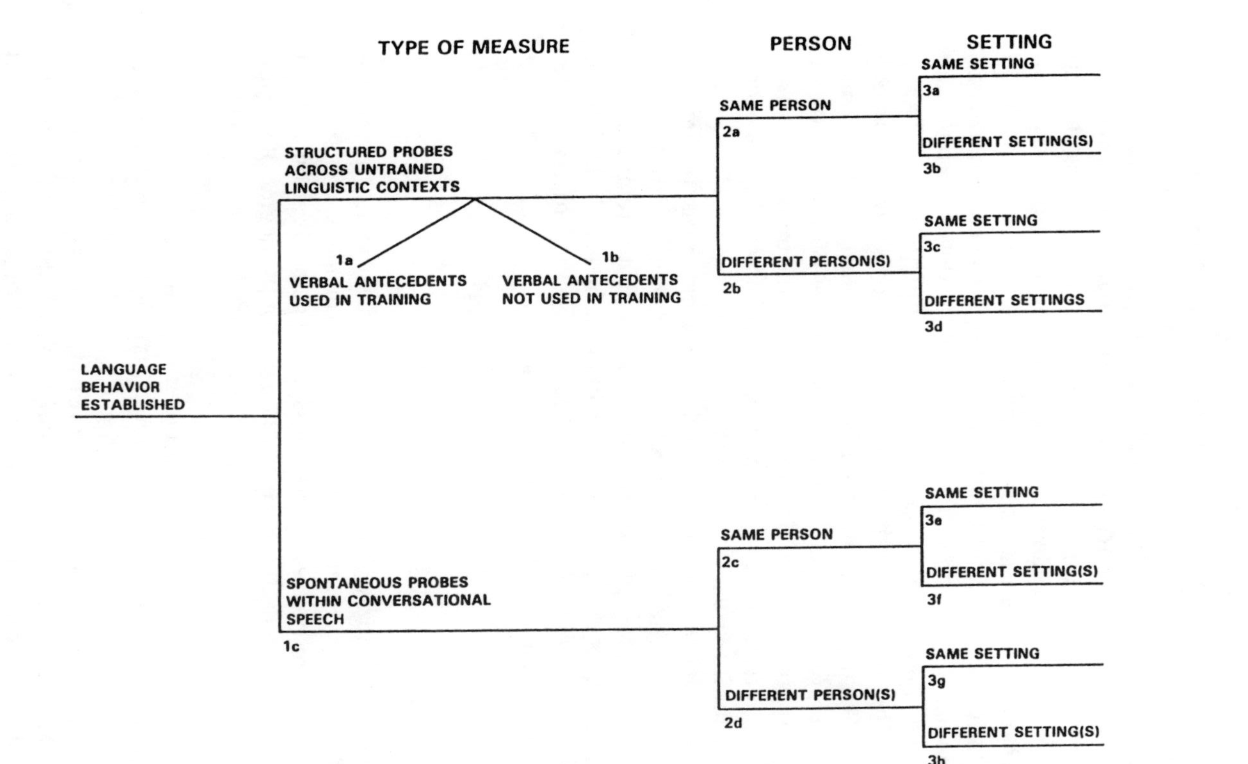

Figure 1–1. Example of some of the varieties of generalization measures. A language behavior established in treatment may be assessed across a number of parameters, including visual and verbal antecedents, persons, and settings, by means of either structured or spontaneous probes.

some aspect of language is produced in linguistic contexts that were not directly trained. This kind of generalization has also been referred to as "intraverbal" generalization (Hegde, 1985). This kind of generalization is particularly crucial for learning the grammatical component of language, since the syntactic and morphological rules must be applied to words and sentences never directly taught in therapy.

The definition of response generalization is not quite as clear-cut as that of stimulus generalization. Response generalization can be conceptualized as finding that the conditioning of one response has influenced the occurrence of a different although related response. For example, after training on sentences such as "The dog is sleeping" and "The bird is flying" to describe pictures, the child produces "The cat is eating." The "different although related response" is clarified in a definition by Warren, Rogers-Warren, Baer, and Guess (1980), which describes response generalization as the display of topographically different responses that are similar in function to the trained responses. For present purposes, the topography of a response can be considered its surface form—visual or auditory.

Response generalization refers to changes in behaviors that are *similar* to, but not the same as, the target behavior (Kazdin, 1980). The more similar a non-reinforced response is to the one that is reinforced, the greater the likelihood of response generalization. Frequently, both stimulus generalization and response generalization occur together, and when the trained behaviors are language behaviors, it is desirable that both co-occur.

Maintenance

Finally, generalization of a trained language structure or response may be measured over time. Usually this is called maintenance. The durability of trained responses is a crucial aspect of generalization and may be a function of the usefulness of the target or of the degree of support for it in the nontraining environment. The nontraining environment itself may have to be changed through the intervention program if the desired language target is to remain over the long run.

Response maintenance may be thought of as the most desirable final goal of any language treatment program. If a client is dismissed from therapy and assessment a year later reveals that the target language behaviors learned in treatment are no longer observable, clinicians need to seriously question their efforts. The thought of such wasted effort should be disheartening to clinicians and clients alike. Maintenance will be further defined and discussed at length in Chapter 7.

EXPLANATIONS FOR GENERALIZATION

While the preceding sections may describe the various phenomena that commonly come under the term generalization, they do not attempt to explain why generalization occurs or fails to occur. Explanations for generalization can be separated into those that emphasize the role of the stimulus and those that emphasize the role of contingencies. As the characteristics of the training stimuli and the generalization stimuli gradually change from greater similarity to less similarity, less generalization may be expected.

The degree of generalization occurring subsequent to training, then, depends on the discrepancy between the crucial characteristics of the training and generalization environments and perhaps on how much discrepancy the individual learner can tolerate. When learners discriminate sufficient differences between the two environments, desired generalization does not occur. Consider two environments, one in which the target behavior receives candy or token reinforcement and one in which no contrived reinforcement is received. When generalization effects are measured, typically no reinforcement is administered; thus, the second environment reflects the "no reinforcement" aspect of natural environments, i.e., the generalization condition. Suppose that after several trials or opportunities the learner no longer produces the target behavior. Discrimination rather than generalization has occurred, and the behavior is extinguished in the generalization condition. In a sense, then, generalization may be viewed as resistance to extinction.

Sometimes, of course, it may be appropriate to discriminate among certain environments and to alter language behaviors accordingly. Thus, whether generalization or discrimination is desirable depends on the particular behavior being taught.

The previous sections provided definitions and discussion of generalization from a behavioral viewpoint. Since most clinicians are familiar with and may use some kind of behavioral paradigm for language intervention, the terminology and framework should be readily assimilated. However, most clinicians are also familiar with a psycholinguistic or cognitive approach to language. A legitimate question at this point would be to ask how non-behaviorists view generalization.

NON-BEHAVIORAL DEFINITIONS OF GENERALIZATION

The generalization problem in language intervention is approached from a different perspective by those who take a more mentalistic or cognitivist view of language. Trained behaviors, such as specific phrase or sentence imitations, may be performed within restricted contexts but remain isolated islands of performance until the child's mental growth allows the formation of a rule. Language forms selected for teaching should be appropriate to the child's level of cognitive development, or they will not enter the child's repertoire as rule-generated language. Some generalization problems may be avoided by increased attention to the interaction between intellectual and linguistic growth. Unfortunately, many of the studies of generalization in language intervention do not report the cognitive levels of the subjects. Behaviorally oriented research may include rough estimates of mental age or functioning age, but not performance on cognitive tasks.

One of the few non-behavioral language researchers to address the problem of generalization in language learning is Johnston (1982). In reviewing the nature of changes in normal language abilities, Johnston described six types of developmental change. These range from the formation of true linguistic categories, as individual lexical elements in multi-word combinations are replaced by more general categorical elements such as nouns and verbs, to the emergence of speaking registers as children learn which words or sentence patterns are appropriate to which listeners, settings, times, topics, and situations. Thus, instead of speaking of setting generalization or generalization across persons, structuralists argue that linguistic behaviors must become "decontextualized" as the language user develops. Certain language aspects must generalize across contexts, and such generalization cannot begin until there is a large enough linguistic repertoire from which to select those that are most appropriate at the moment.

The problem of getting trained grammatical targets to generalize to spontaneous production is viewed by Johnston (1982) as automatization, a process "... fundamentally different than generalization" (p. 50). Apparently, neither normal children nor language-disordered children master grammatical morpheme rules in one fell swoop. There is a period of time over which the use of grammatical morphemes gradually becomes more consistent. According to Brown's longitudinal study of normal children, "... a considerable period of time elapses between the first appearance of a morpheme and the point where it is almost always supplied where required" (Brown, 1973, p. 257). He goes on to say that this fact "... does not accord well with the notion that the acquisition of grammar is a matter of the acquisition of rules...," in which case "One would expect rule acquisition to be sudden" (p. 257). For a while, performance factors (e.g., familiarity with vocabulary items, complexity of linguistic context, and degree of propositionality of the utterance) seem to affect the production of particular morphemes at any one time. As greater demand is placed on the child's attentional resources, rules that have not become automatic may not be applied. With repeated practice, however, production of most grammatical morphemes becomes habitual.

According to Johnston, then, there are two distinct generalization problems. One is the child with narrow rules, who requires specific additional instances of linguistic data from which to figure out the more general rule. The other is the child who applies a rule inconsistently, probably owing to performance constraints, who needs graded opportunities to practice production of rule-governed sentences (Johnston, 1982). Rather than investigate such behavioral phenomena as factors in the stimulus complex that affect setting generalization or person generalization or the composition of various language response classes, structuralists would urge that a careful description of the child's prior linguistic (and cognitive) knowledge is necessary before investigations begin to focus on the number of exemplars needed to infer a general rule or the best sequence in which to train a rule.

SUMMARY

This chapter was designed to establish the scope of the term *generalization* for this book. By now the reader should be familiar with some of the jargon of the generalization literature. Perhaps some of those terms will find their way into lesson plans, treatment programs, or discussions with co-teachers.

Three categories to describe the occurrence of generalization within language intervention were presented. After a period of treatment, generalization might occur spontaneously, without any direct efforts to achieve it. More likely, generalization measures may indicate that the language target has failed to generalize across one or several parameters. In this case, a specially designed generalization phase of the treatment program may be applied post-hoc and result in generalization. Alternatively, treatment programs may be designed to forestall generalization failure and include strategies to promote generalization across various parameters very early in the treatment program.

The various parameters of the stimulus complex were described as part of the concept of stimulus generalization. The parameters of verbal and visual antecedents, persons, and settings were explored as possible factors that may be associated with generalization failure. Response generalization was described as a major feature of language learning, since the grammatical component of language requires that rules be learned that will result in production of novel utterances not directly taught in therapy. Finally, maintenance was introduced as the ultimate goal of language intervention.

While generalization is most often viewed from a behavioral perspective, those who view language from a mentalistic or cognitive perspective have also used the term. What may be viewed as a failure of the language target to generalize across persons, settings, and verbal or visual antecedents may also be described as the failure of a language production mechanism to reach an "automatic" level.

Although various researchers and clinicians may define the concept more narrowly, a broader, more inclusive definition of generalization will be used within this book. As future research reveals more about the nature of the phenomenon called *generalization*, more precise terms will come into use for various aspects of it.

Chapter 2

Measurement of Generalization

Whether the clinician programs for generalization from the beginning of treatment or establishes the target and then checks for generalization, the language intervention program must provide for measurements of generalization of the target language behaviors. The concern of this chapter is how and when to measure the various kinds of generalization accurately and efficiently and how to interpret the results of such measures.

TYPES OF GENERALIZATION MEASURES

To monitor the kinds and amounts of generalization that are occurring during the intervention process, at least two types of measures are advisable: structured probes and spontaneous probes. A structured probe is similar to treatment conditions, except for the parameters being checked. An unstructured, spontaneous probe checks for generalization of target behaviors or skills to real use in natural environments, which differ considerably from treatment conditions. Both types of generalization measures have been described by Connell (1982) and Warren, Rogers-Warren, Baer, and Guess (1980).

Structured Probes of Generalization

Structured probe measures of generalization may be thought of as small tests to see whether a language target that has been learned to some performance criterion in treatment is produced under some new conditions. Measurement occurs within situations where the stimulus and response characteristics are similar to the ones used in training; only one or two parameters of the training situation are different. For instance, picture cards used in therapy are sent home to be presented by a parent in a structured format similar to that used in therapy, but with no reinforcement for correct responding. Results of such a probe would reveal whether setting and person generalization has occurred.

Another example of a structured probe for generalization of a language target would be the presentation by the clinician in a therapy session of new pictures or other stimuli that require a particular grammatical structure for description. After the grammatical rule has been learned in treatment using a practiced set of pictures, a set of unpracticed pictures is used to determine whether the rule can be extended to new examples. The semantic content of the sentence descriptions would be new (unpracticed), but the syntactic or morphological structure would be the learned response that has (or has not) generalized. The degree of structure and the verbal antecedents used in these probes are generally similar to those of the treatment sessions. Performance in response to these unpracticed stimuli can indicate the first stages of generalization, which would probably not be evident in conversational language measures.

Most experimental studies have relied solely on structured probes to assess generalization of language targets. Structured generalization probes have been collected in nontraining settings, have employed different persons, and have utilized stimuli that differed in some way from those used in training. Table 2–1 summarizes a number of these operant studies that employed structured generalization probes.

While combining several of these parameters may make structured probes of generalization somewhat similar to the measurement of generalization to spontaneous production in natural environments, this kind of generalization measure is essentially more structured, more like treatment, than other measures. Therefore, generalization as measured by structured probes may occur more quickly and easily than generalization measured by spontaneous probes.

Spontaneous Probes of Generalization

Even though structured probes of language target generalization may show correct production across several parameters (e.g., verbal and visual antecedents, persons, and settings), the target may still be produced incorrectly (or not at all) in spontaneous, conversational language. It seems as though the client can "remember to say it right" when there is some structure that provides a cue to do so, but "forgets" when formulating sentences to communicate ideas without any reminders to pay attention to form. Thus, a crucial generalization measure is some observational probe of communicative language behavior in unstructured, nontreatment environments.

The results of spontaneous probes can show whether the language target(s) have generalized to the natural environment. Warren and coworkers (1980) used the term *natural environment generalization* for

Table 2–1. Operant Studies that Employed Structured Generalization Probes

Authors	Subjects	Language Target	Generalization
Garcia (1974)	2 MR adolescents	Answers to questions: "It is a ________" and "Yes, I do"	To three nontraining settings and adults; reinforcement needed in two of the settings
Martin (1975)	2 MR children	Color and size adjectives: [adjective + N]	To two nontraining settings and adults and to untrained items in response to nontraining stimuli
Rubin and Stolz (1974)	1 MR adolescent	Pronouns and self-referent speech: [*I, my, you, your, she, he* + N]	To untrained combinations in response to teacher's training questions in the classroom
Wheeler and Sulzer (1970)	1 speech-deficient child	Complete sentences: [N + *is* + V + *-ing*]	To untrained items in response to verbal stimuli used in training
Hegde, Noll, and Pecora (1975)	2 language-delayed children	Pronouns [*he, she, it*], auxiliary and copular [*'s, was*], and possessive [*'s -s/-z*]	To untrained items in response to verbal stimuli used in training and to mother at home (for 1 child)
Twardosz and Baer (1973)	2 MR adolescents	*wh-* questions: "What [color, letter, number]?"	To untrained items in response to presentation of card and no verbal stimuli
Bennett and Ling (1972)	1 hearing-impaired child	Complete sentences: [*The* N + *is* + V + *-ing*]	To untrained items in response to verbal stimuli used in training
Clark and Sherman (1975)	3 MR adolescents and 4 disadvantaged children	Past and future tense and verb participle	To untrained items in response to verbal stimuli used in training
Garcia, Guess, and Byrnes (1973)	1 MR child	Singular and plural sentences: "That is one ________" and "These are two ________"	To untrained items in response to verbal stimuli used in training
Lutzker and Sherman (1974)	3 MR and 4 normal subjects	Subject-verb agreement: [N + *(s)* + *is/are* + V + *-ing*]	To untrained sentences in response to verbal stimuli used in training
Schumaker and Sherman (1970)	3 MR adolescents	Past tense and progressive verb usage	To untrained items in response to verbal stimuli used in training

this kind of generalization, which is assessed by observing the client under unstructured, nontraining conditions as he or she spontaneously produces language in response to the varied stimuli that occur outside the treatment environment.

The language observed could be the trained language (e.g., vocabulary, multi-word phrases), a combination of trained and untrained language forms (e.g., grammatical morphemes or syntactic constructions), or novel productions that were not directly trained (e.g., a trained grammatical construction with untrained content words). The evaluator makes no specific attempts to elicit the target response from the child, since listeners in the natural environment may not do so. For example, an observer records language samples of the client during a free-play period in the classroom, and productions of the language target when appropriate opportunities occur are noted. Even during a therapy session, a clinician may have an opportunity to measure this kind of generalization, for example, when spontaneous conversational language is produced before and after structured teaching tasks or as the client is entering or leaving the therapy room.

The majority of language generalization studies have not reported measures of this kind, or if they do, details concerning measurement procedures are sparse; for example, the verbal antecedents of language targets are seldom reported. There are several reasons for such infrequent reports of natural environment generalization. For one thing, assessing generalization in the natural environment requires considerable time for observation and analysis. For another, clinical researchers may have assumed that generalization to the natural environment would occur automatically after structured probes reveal generalization across several parameters, and so did not check for it.

It is far easier to measure generalization of language targets to untrained exemplars, settings, or persons using structured probes than it is to measure generalization to language produced and understood in the natural environment or maintained there. While natural-environment generalization may be the most important kind to assess, it may be a difficult measure to arrange. Audio or video tape recordings of clients in several natural environments may be necessary to measure natural-environment generalization unobtrusively. Indeed, it could be argued that such recordings are not unobtrusive. Just as children may realize when they are being tested and produce trained language, clients may realize that an observer or recorder is present and adjust language performance accordingly.

A lengthy sample or multiple samples may be needed to ensure that several opportunities to produce the language targets occur. Time-sampling procedures have been used by some investigators, whereas others have collected short samples by verbatim transcription in vivo, supplemented by tape recordings obtained via a transmitter worn by the child (Hughes, 1982; Warren et al., 1980). Natural environments have included the child's home and various school settings, such as regular classrooms and free-play time.

Difficult though it may be to assess, natural-environment generalization is undoubtedly the ultimate test of the effectiveness of the language intervention program. The most rigorous measure of generalization would occur under conditions that are extremely different from the treatment conditions. Unfortunately, the more rigorous the method of assessment, the more disappointing the results are likely to be (Forehand and Atkeson, 1977). However, failure on such rigorous tests of generalization should result in changes in the intervention program such that the training and natural environments gradually become more similar.

Even though production of a language target in spontaneous conversational speech may not be an immediate goal of intervention, it may be a good idea to keep this "ultimate test" of successful language intervention in mind from the beginning of therapy. For one thing, it may influence the clinician's choice of target—pick something that has a good chance of being needed in conversational production and that is simple and easy enough to be taught in a reasonably short time. For another thing, taking a baseline measure of conversational language production, if the conversation occurs with a frequent listener in the child's nontreatment environment, can provide the clinician with some idea of how that listener's language could be altered to facilitate generalization of a target language behavior. Thus, some initial measure of conversational production can serve several useful purposes as well as providing a baseline against which to compare progress after some period of treatment.

Perhaps it should be mentioned here that for clients who do not produce intelligible spoken language, the conversational sample may require the presence of conversational partners who sign or interact via communication boards. This may be the clinician or some other person. The important aspect is the nontreatment nature of the sample—the client's spontaneous use of his or her language system for communicative purposes in nontreatment situations must be observed.

Maintenance Probes

A third kind of generalization measure proposed by Warren and colleagues (1980) is *maintenance*, or generalization across time. This differs from natural-environment generalization in that the effects of training are measured by either structured or natural environment probes after all formal intervention has ceased (Warren et al., 1980). Maintenance also implies that a substantial period has elapsed between termination of treatment and follow-up measures.

The crucial factor in measuring this form of generalization is whether treatment is considered ongoing or terminated (Drabman, Hammer, and Rosenbaum, 1979). Treatment may be considered ongoing if any programmatic contingencies controlled by teacher or therapist remain in effect. Under this definition, maintenance of language behaviors may be assessed within natural environments, which may include planned opportunities for display of the language target as long as no contingencies are applied.

In their research on autistic children, Koegel and Rincover (1977) distinguished between generalization and maintenance of behaviors in extra-therapy settings after initial acquisition in therapy. The three children studied learned the behaviors in therapy and maintained them there. Two of the children generalized the behavior to the extra-therapy setting, but the behavior was not maintained there. Apparently, once reinforcing contingencies were removed, the behavior gradually extinguished. The third child did not generalize the behavior to the extra-therapy setting. Thus, separate deficits in generalization and maintenance were measured.

Measures of maintenance, then, must involve both a time-lapse between treatment termination and the maintenance measure and the absence of contingencies from the treatment program. For example, after successful generalization of a language target to spontaneous production in the natural environment has occurred and training on that target has ceased, three-month and six-month maintenance probes are conducted. Although treatment for other language targets may continue, therapy for the language target in question has been discontinued.

MEASURING GENERALIZATION BY STRUCTURED AND SPONTANEOUS PROBES

Structured probes using nontraining exemplars have been used in a number of controlled operant studies of the generalization of grammatical or syntactic targets to untrained linguistic contexts (Hegde, 1980; Hegde, Noll, and Pecora, 1979; Hegde and Gierut, 1979). Typically, an interspersed (intermixed) trial procedure is used, which allows responses to the nontraining stimuli to go unreinforced. Prior to the structured probe, the practiced, training stimuli have been reinforced on a fixed or variable-ratio schedule; therefore, interspersing new stimuli with old stimuli allows this schedule to be continued for the structured probes. In this way, generalization of the target to untrained linguistic contexts required by the new stimuli can be measured. This interspersing procedure also minimizes the possibility that subjects will discriminate between training and probe trials. When a block of untrained probe stimuli are presented, the behavior may readily extinguish because of the lack of contingent reinforcement.

Since generalization of language behaviors can occur along a number of parameters or combinations of them (e.g., visual stimuli, verbal antecedents, persons, settings), measurement of the amount of generalization that has occurred subsequent to a period of treatment can vary along a number of parameters also. Both structured and spontaneous probes can be used to assess generalization across these parameters. Controlled studies of generalization often choose only one or two parameters to measure, so that effects of a particular training program on any one parameter can be observed. Clinically, however, it would not be desirable to measure or program for only one parameter at a time.

The following sections present issues in measuring generalization across the parameters of visual and verbal antecedents, persons, and settings. Examples from experimental studies will be included to illustrate methods of measuring generalization.

Probes of Nontreatment Verbal and Visual Antecedents

Often, language teaching programs have built into them a progression of verbal antecedents, e.g., "Tell me: (model of target)," followed by some kind of *wh-* question such as "What are they doing?" and finally some general directive such as "Tell me about them." Thus, some assessment of generalization across verbal antecedents may be done as the clinician moves through various steps of the teaching program.

While this hierarchy of verbal antecedents may successfully result in production of target responses, it may also trigger the child's awareness of a generalization test. Clinicians are often advised to use "Tell me about..." and "Tell me some more" in collecting spontaneous language samples. If these phrases have also been used in the treatment program, it seems likely that they would serve to remind the child to use a particular language target and thus would not provide a representative sample of true generalization to natural environments.

In their study of generalization of a syntax target following application of an operant remediation program (the Monterey Program), Mulac and Tomlinson (1977) used a variety of verbal antecedents to evoke *is*-interrogatives in an extended transfer program. For example, a few sentences of a story were read to the child, and then the book was hidden from him or her. The adult then looked at a page and said, "I see a bird. Guess if the bird is flying or sleeping." For pre-treatment and post-treatment language samples, a set of six language collection tasks ranging from immediate imitation to talk in free play was administered. Tasks included such verbal antecedents as "We can't open the box until you guess what's inside. Guess what's in the box" or "I feel something in the bag. Is it an airplane? No. Is it a ball? Yes, it's a ball. Now it's your turn."

Results of this study indicated that subjects improved more on some of the six language tasks than others. Specifically, tasks using more structured verbal antecedents such as "... Guess what's in the box" or "... Now it's your turn." were more likely to elicit correct *is*-interrogatives than were tasks using less structured verbal antecedents such as "... Let's play" or "I'm going to give you this piece of candy in three minutes."

This study illustrates the importance of the verbal antecedents used in collecting generalization data. It would be interesting to know if the correct *is*-questions would have occurred on unobtrusive observational measures that did not include deliberate tasks for evoking them. On one hand, providing verbal antecedents that are known to provide opportunities for display of the target makes the generalization measure more efficient, but on the other hand, it limits the kinds of generalization that can be observed.

Visual stimuli to be used during generalization assessment may also present a dilemma. An efficient probe would use visual stimuli likely to evoke the target, but if these stimuli have been used in treatment, then they cannot reveal generalization across visual antecedents.

Language training often begins with the teaching of object labels, nouns representing common objects. Several studies of early language teaching have indicated that objects are better than pictures as teaching stimuli, at least for some learners (Olswang, Bain, Dunn, and Cooper, 1983; Welch and Pear, 1980). Even when objects are used, however, it is necessary that labels be applied to several examples of an object (large and small balls, metal and plastic spoons); otherwise, it is doubtful that a semantic concept has been formed for the word. Eventually, it will be more efficient to teach vocabulary by using pictures rather than objects; therefore, it is also necessary that children generalize labels from objects to pictures and vice versa.

Person Probes

Measures of language target generalization across persons (listeners, conversational partners) may involve structured probes or spontaneous probes and may or may not include the visual and verbal antecedents used in treatment. An early and simple person probe may include bringing a child's parent or sibling into the therapy session. Asking a classroom teacher or teacher's aide to administer a structured probe can also provide a measure of generalization across persons. If a peer has been used in the treatment program, a generalization measure should be taken without that peer present. In measuring generalization across persons, the crucial element to vary is the person (clinician, parent, peer) who has administered the treatment.

When arranging for a person not involved in treatment to collect generalization data, some instruction will be necessary. If child-initiated communicative language is a target, it is crucial that the listeners in the generalization setting be cautioned to wait long enough to allow such language from the client. Ideally, the data collector should not be aware of the language target nor be familiar with treatment procedures, especially for a spontaneous probe. A tape recorder turned on during dinnertime conversation may be used to collect a spontaneous language sample for noting generalized behaviors, or a tape recording of the child playing or looking at books with an older sibling may result in a sample for generalization assessment. For social language behaviors, such as greetings and closings, or social initiations, an observer may hand-record brief samples at specific times during the day.

In collecting measures of generalization across persons, the typical listeners available to the client should be considered as conversation partners or data collectors. However, the same language behaviors may not be appropriate for use with all listeners. Since adjustments in language based on the person addressed is part of pragmatic language competence, the clinician must consider whether or not the target language is appropriate for use with particular listeners used for the generalization measure.

Setting Probes

Like measures of person generalization, measures of setting generalization can be carried out by using either structured or spontaneous probes and may or may not include persons and visual or verbal antecedents used in treatment. Perhaps the simplest test of setting generalization would be for the clinician to use the training stimuli (verbal and visual) in a nontherapy room within the school or clinic. If correct responding occurs at a level similar to that found in the therapy room, generalization across one setting has occurred. Additional settings (home, playground, gym, bus, car) may be employed to check for generalization across several settings. Some investigators have employed a narrower definition of "setting" than others—e.g., different rooms within one building versus multiple buildings or outdoor locations. Research by Handleman (1979, 1981) included measures of generalization within several places in the training center and also within the child's home.

The clinician seeking to measure setting generalization faces several decisions. In what locations is it reasonable to expect and test for generalization? Who will carry out generalization probes? What verbal and visual antecedents, if any, should be used? If the client lives in a sheltered environment—institution, group home, with parents—this should certainly be considered as a place to assess language generalization. If a child rides a bus to and from school or stays with a babysitter or at a day-care center part of the day, then these are probably places where the language targets should be displayed. Consider the client's daily or weekly routine, and several important settings in which to measure generalization should come to mind.

The decision regarding who should carry out setting generalization measures may be answered by default, i.e., who is *willing* to do it? However, given that choices of people exist, there may be two disadvantages to the training clinician carrying out the setting generalization measure. First, if the clinician happens to be the controlling stimulus for the language target and he or she is not usually in the generalization setting, success on the probe would give false hope—the desired language would not occur in the setting unless the clinician also was there. Second, the measure would only reveal setting generalization, when perhaps both person and setting generalization have occurred. Clinically, it would be more efficient to assess two parameters than one. Nevertheless, someone must carry out the structured probe in the nontraining settings, and if no one else will do it then that task may fall to the clinician.

If the setting generalization probe is to be a spontaneous probe, then an observer who will not interact with the client is needed. Studies done in a university setting often utilize undergraduate or graduate students to observe and record behaviors after some training in what and how to observe. This is probably a luxury available to few practicing clinicians. In school settings, perhaps upper-grade students could be recruited for such observation, or parents or siblings of the client may be persuaded to collect some data. In institutional settings, perhaps some of the ward staff may be helpful, or if other professional services are available, perhaps a cooperative effort can be mounted to observe several behaviors.

Whether the setting generalization is measured by a non-clinician using a structured probe or by a non-clinician observing language behaviors in the natural environment, some training should be given to the data collector. The simpler the data collection procedure is, the more reliable it will be and the more likely it will be completed. Brief training that includes practice in scoring or observing should be carried out. However, there is always the possibility of observer bias, especially within natural environment checks, and attention should be given to this issue.

WHEN TO ASSESS FOR GENERALIZATION

It may be that generalization of some language targets to spontaneous production in natural environments will not occur until well after the targets have successfully generalized on structured probes across several parameters. Generalized responses to the structured stimuli used in such probes may be a necessary prerequisite to generalized production in natural environments (Warren et al., 1980). However, at present controlled comparison studies between structured probe generalization and spontaneous natural-environment generalization have rarely been reported. For one study of generalization subsequent to language treatment in four nonretarded language-impaired children, both structured probes in the treatment setting and spontaneous probes in the children's homes were collected before and during treatment (Hughes, 1982). Comparisons of correct production of the grammatical targets (*is* and *are*) as they occurred on structured and spontaneous probes revealed that structured probe scores were higher than spontaneous probe scores when data for *is* and *are* were combined, as shown in Figure 2–1.

These data support the assumption made by Warren and colleagues, but more empirical research with varied populations and language targets is required before the assumption can be taken as fact.

For most language intervention, structured probe measures for checking generalization across settings, persons, and untrained exemplars should probably precede spontaneous probes of natural-environment generalization. It may be that some clients' language behaviors will never meet that most rigorous test of generalization, observation of communicative language in natural environments. Indeed, the goal for some clients may be only to achieve generalization of trained language target behaviors within a supportive environment, i.e., one that has been altered to ensure numerous opportunities to produce the desired language targets and to reinforce them when they occur.

HOW STRUCTURED IS "STRUCTURED"?

Conditions under which measurement occurs are usually quite clearly and easily defined as different from treatment conditions. A setting either was or was not used for treatment. A person either was or was not involved in training the targets. Specific visual or verbal stimuli either were or were not used during training. However, there is another aspect of generalization measurement that is not so clearly dichotomous, i.e., the degree of structure imposed on the language produced during treatment and generalization sessions. The variety of language produced by both the client and the listener during the therapy sessions and during the generalization measures may not be easily described dichotomously as "structured" or "unstructured." Rather, such language may be placed along a continuum from "highly structured" to "loosely structured."

To illustrate this point, consider the following example. During diagnostic evaluations of children who have been in treatment, clinicians may notice a "rehearsed" quality in the language samples collected from certain children. With or without prompting, for example, the child may produce a set of present progressive sentences with *is* stressed while

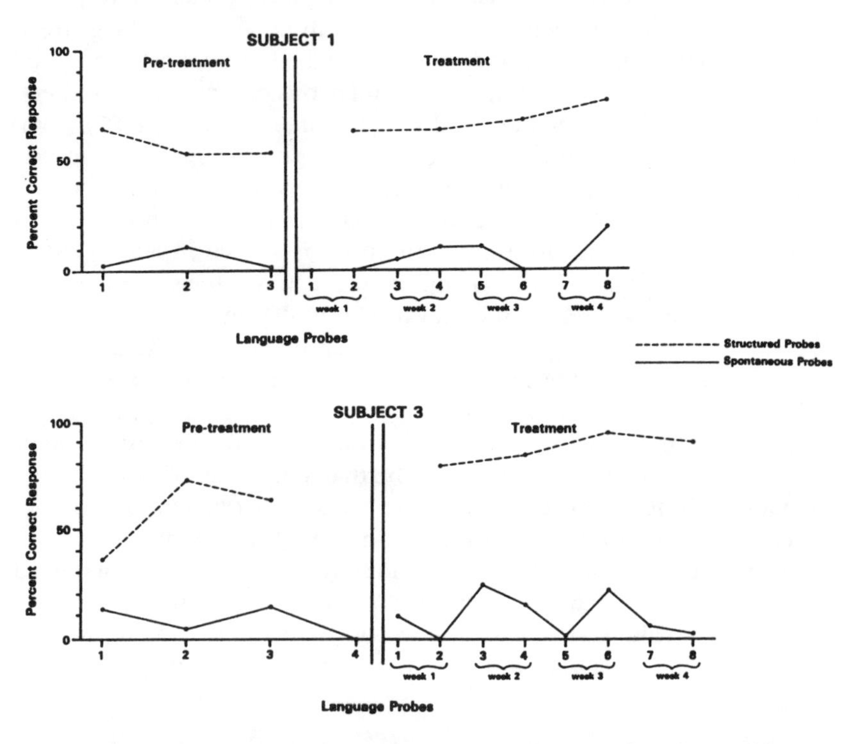

Figure 2–1. Discrepancies between scores on structured probes and spontaneous probe scores for production of *is* and *are* from four language-impaired children.

playing with toys or may produce a descriptive sentence that includes a specific morpheme for every page in a book. The diagnostic clinician concludes, probably correctly, that the child has realized that a test is occurring and is deliberately producing language targets previously trained or currently emphasized in therapy. Since the setting, listener, and quite likely the materials differ from those present during treatment, the conclusion can be drawn that some desirable generalization across several parameters has occurred. But clinicians are also aware of the conscious, rehearsed quality of this language and rightly wonder if the grammar targets would occur when the child talks in a nontest situation.

As the previous example illustrates, changes in some parameters of the treatment conditions can indicate that some generalization has occurred, but additional instances of those same changes may not yield similar results. In how many nontreatment settings, or with how many nontreatment listeners, will the trained language target be displayed? Will it sound deliberate and rehearsed? Or will it sound like normal con-

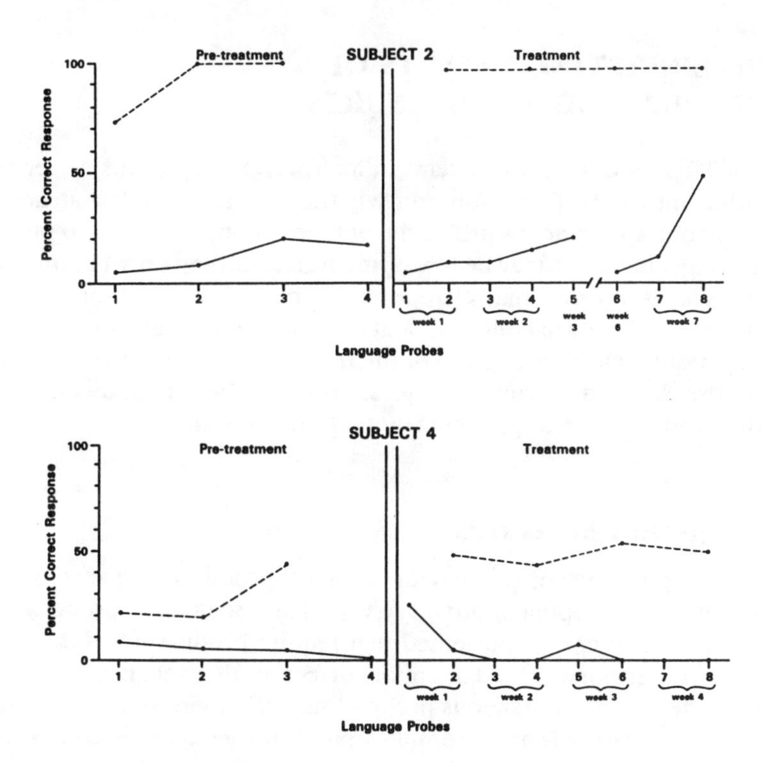

Figure 2–1. (continued).

versational speech? Will this depend on the degree of structure of the generalization measure?

Again, the similarity between treatment and generalization conditions is crucial. If the generalization measure is highly structured—for example, a block of ten questions—and the treatment format has been highly structured, then the likelihood of correct responding is increased. When treatment consists of massed trial training, where 10 or 20 items are practiced as a block, structured probe generalization may be readily achieved. However, suppose the generalization measure is an observation of 10 or 20 opportunities to produce the target dispersed throughout a day. Under these conditions, correct production may rarely occur. The discrepancy between treatment and generalization conditions may be too great. Indeed, several authors have suggested that treatment formats should rely more on dispersed or distributed trial training, thus making treatment and generalization conditions similar (McCormick and Schiefelbusch, 1984; McLean, Snyder-McLean, and Sack, 1981).

INTERPRETING RESULTS OF GENERALIZATION MEASURES

There are several problems in interpreting the results of generalization measures. Depending on whether the measure is a structured probe or a spontaneous probe, the number of opportunities to produce the target behavior may be few or many. Depending on what the target behavior is, the data may change in unexpected ways as more generalization measures are collected. Making sense of the generalization data may require close inspection of the results of generalization measures. For the clinician, a prominent question should be kept in focus: "Is this kind and amount of generalization clinically significant?"

Frequency Measures

Suppose the target behavior is correct production of sentences requiring *is* as a copula or auxiliary verb. For a structured probe, a number of stimuli can be presented that require production of the target, and a straightforward judgment of correct or incorrect production can be made. For a spontaneous probe of natural-environment generalization, the measure is more complicated. If the behavior desired is spontaneous production, then specific planned opportunities to elicit the target behavior should not be used. However, if no opportunities are planned, there is a risk of getting no target behaviors, because no natural opportunities occurred. This would result in a 0/0 fraction, which should not be interpreted as 0 per cent correct occurrence. Since there are no data for that particular generalization session, a gap will occur in the series of generalization measures. This points out the importance of repeated measures of generalization. If only one post-treatment measure is obtained for natural-environment generalization, there may be no data to show whether or not generalization has occurred.

The problem of infrequent natural opportunities continues when only two, three, or four opportunities occur. Suppose that for five generalization measures, the following numbers of opportunities occur: 5, 2, 3, 1, and 3, and that for each measure the target was correctly produced only once. The following percentages of correct productions would result: 20 per cent, 50 per cent, 33 per cent, 100 per cent, 33 per cent. How would the clinician interpret these results? If the data were presented in absolute frequencies of occurrence, a flat graph would result, but a jagged profile would result from the percentage data. Clearly, a difference in interpretation of results can result from the form in which data are presented.

Sometimes frequency data are reported in multiples of the baseline values. For example, Strain (1977) reported a fivefold increase in the frequency of positive social behaviors initiated by two children during treatment sessions, whereas generalization data showed only twice the level observed during baseline measures. How should these data be interpreted? Should the frequency of the target behavior be the same in treatment and in generalization sessions? For social initiations, probably not. For production of grammatically correct sentences, however, the target structure should be produced whenever an obligatory context occurs. Thus, the nature of the target behavior can influence the interpretation of generalization data.

When the generalization data measured involve a grammatical form, another problem arises in data collection. If the form can occur in several different sentence types, should data include production in all the available obligatory contexts or only in the sentence types trained? For example, yes-no questions such as "Is it raining?" and "Is it red?" require *is*, but in the initial position rather than following the subject. If baseline measures have indicated that *is* is in error in both sentence positions, generalization data collected on all *is* productions may reveal some patterns of response class formation.

Duration Versus Frequency

One final example of problems in interpreting generalization measures is illustrated by the results of a study by Hendrickson, Strain, Tremblay, and Shores (1982). These investigators measured the frequency of social initiations, such as "Let's play house," and responses to initiations by children in a playroom. During an initial phase of treatment, initiations increased, as anticipated. However, during a second treatment phase, the frequency of initiations decreased. A straightforward interpretation of the data would result in the conclusion that the second treatment phase was not effective. By looking at the *durations* of each social exchange, however, it was apparent that the exchanges in the second phase were twice as long as those of the first phase. Thus, as the duration of social exchanges increased, the need for many initiations decreased, explaining the reduced frequency of social initiations during the second treatment phase. In terms of verbal social behavior, longer exchanges are more desirable than frequent short ones, so the outcome of this treatment was positive. If careful analysis of the data had not been done, the results of the measures could easily have been misinterpreted.

Clinically Significant Generalization

Quite often, generalization measures do not reveal 100 per cent generalization of a target behavior across the desired parameter(s). In some cases, production of a few examples of the target behavior under nontreatment conditions may be sufficient for the clinician to believe that *some* generalization is occurring. In assessing setting generalization by a transfer test of ten trials, Rincover and Koegel (1975) found a low of 30 per cent and a high of 80 per cent generalization of the trained behavior for six of the ten autistic children who had reached treatment criterion. Interestingly, all six responded correctly on the first trial presented in the new setting, i.e., before they could know that no food or praise would be given for correct responding. The remaining four children showed no generalization. In interpreting this data, it is appropriate to ask whether 30 per cent correct responding is clinically significant generalization. At what point can it be concluded that generalization has occurred? Reliance on only one measure of generalization is dangerous; it would also be important to determine what performance would be observed on several additional generalization measures.

Determination of clinical significance is closely connected with the kinds of measures used and the kind of target behavior chosen. For language behaviors that are not required to occur 100 per cent of the time, the frequency with which normal language users produce the behavior may be used as a guide for determining how frequently the generalized behavior should occur. For example, labeling statements such as "That's a horse" may not occur very frequently in natural environments, except when directly requested. Requests for objects or actions may occur only when an internal need exists and help from another person is desired for meeting that need. Children who can help themselves probably do not use verbal requests as often as handicapped children. Production of two- and three-word utterances that express early semantic relations, such as "mommy eat cookie" or "cookie fall floor," need not occur every time an appropriate opportunity occurs. Thus, when generalization of such targets is measured, a criterion level of 50 per cent correct responding to appropriate verbal and nonverbal events may be considered a clinically significant level of generalization. As an alternative, the clinician may also decide to use a 50 per cent increase over baseline levels as a criterion measure for successful generalization. For experimental research, a social validation measure may be obtained by assessing the rate or frequency of the language target behavior within normal dyads or groups (Gajar, Schloss, Schloss, and Thompson, 1984).

Grammatical language targets, on the other hand, must be used in nearly 100 per cent of their obligatory linguistic contexts if the speaker is to appear normal. Indeed, normal speakers who occasionally produce ungrammatical sentences (e.g., "He don't have none" or "I seen it") are said to use bad grammar. When Brown studied the acquisition of his famous 14 grammatical morphemes, he used as the criterion for acquisition occurrence of the morpheme in 90 per cent of the obligatory contexts found in the language samples. For these grammatical language behaviors, then, 90 to 100 per cent correct responding may be necessary if generalization is to be considered clinically significant.

WITHIN-SUBJECT EXPERIMENTAL DESIGNS

Many of the studies that will be summarized in the following chapters used within-subject (single-subject) experimental designs to investigate the generalization effects of various language treatment programs. These designs were specifically developed to explore the effectiveness of events in treating disordered populations (Kazdin, 1982; McReynolds and Kearns, 1983), and they are especially powerful in examining generalization issues. Since some readers may not be familiar with these designs, brief descriptions of the more common ones are provided here. For readers interested in more detail, the book *Single-Subject Experimental Designs in Communicative Disorders* (McReynolds and Kearns, 1983) is highly recommended.

Multiple-baseline designs are within-subject experimental designs that require repeated measurement of some variables that do *not* receive treatment, as well as repeated measurement of the treated variable. The variables can be particular behavioral responses (e.g., language targets), the subjects themselves, or settings and persons across which generalization is desired. For example, a multiple-baseline design across behaviors might use three manual signs, for example, *cookie, milk, apple.* Baseline levels of production would be established for all three signs, then treatment would begin on *cookie* while continued measurement of production of all three signs occurs periodically, for example, with weekly probes. If treatment results in improved production of the treated sign, while production of the untreated signs remains low, then the clinical researcher can conclude that improvement was the result of treatment and not of time or maturation, which would have affected the other behaviors. The stability of the second and third baselines demonstrates that treatment affects only the behavior to which it is applied.

After improvement is shown for the first sign, treatment is applied to the second sign while baseline measures continue for the third sign. Change in the second sign must be similar to that shown for the first sign, although it may take fewer sessions or trials to meet criterion. Treatment on the third sign begins after improvement is shown for the second sign. Thus, each untreated sign has served a control function for the experiment.

The need for this control feature means that automatic or spontaneous generalization should not occur, or the multiple-baseline control will be lost. Thus, independence of various behaviors, settings, or persons must be assumed. However, generalization measures in nontreatment settings or with nontreatment persons may be taken along with the continued baseline probes in treatment settings. In this way, treatment effects within generalization conditions may be monitored during a multiple-baseline experiment.

The behaviors monitored and subsequently treated in a multiple-baseline design across behaviors may be grammatical targets, and generalization measures may include production of those targets within untrained linguistic contexts (sentences). Figure 2–2 illustrates effects of a treatment program for grammar targets applied first to production of the subject pronoun *she*, then to the subject pronoun *it*, and finally to the auxiliary or copular verb *are*. These hypothetical data show training only on the first two sentences for each target, but more sentences may be needed before the desired generalization is achieved.

Withdrawal and reversal designs provide a convincing demonstration of experimental control over the occurrence and nonoccurrence of target behaviors, thus allowing assessment of cause and effect relationships. Typically, a four-phase A-B-A-B design is used, in which A represents no treatment or reversal of treatment, and B represents treatment. After an initial baseline is established, treatment is applied until a certain criterion is reached. Then the treatment is either withdrawn or reversed. An example of reversing a behavior would be to train *omission* of *is* in sentences after treatment had resulted in inclusion of this morpheme. Experimental control is shown as behavior rates change with application and withdrawal or reversal of treatment, indicating that change was functionally related to treatment.

The example of an A-B-A-B design shown in Figure 2–3 illustrates effects of a role-playing treatment program for initiating requests, with

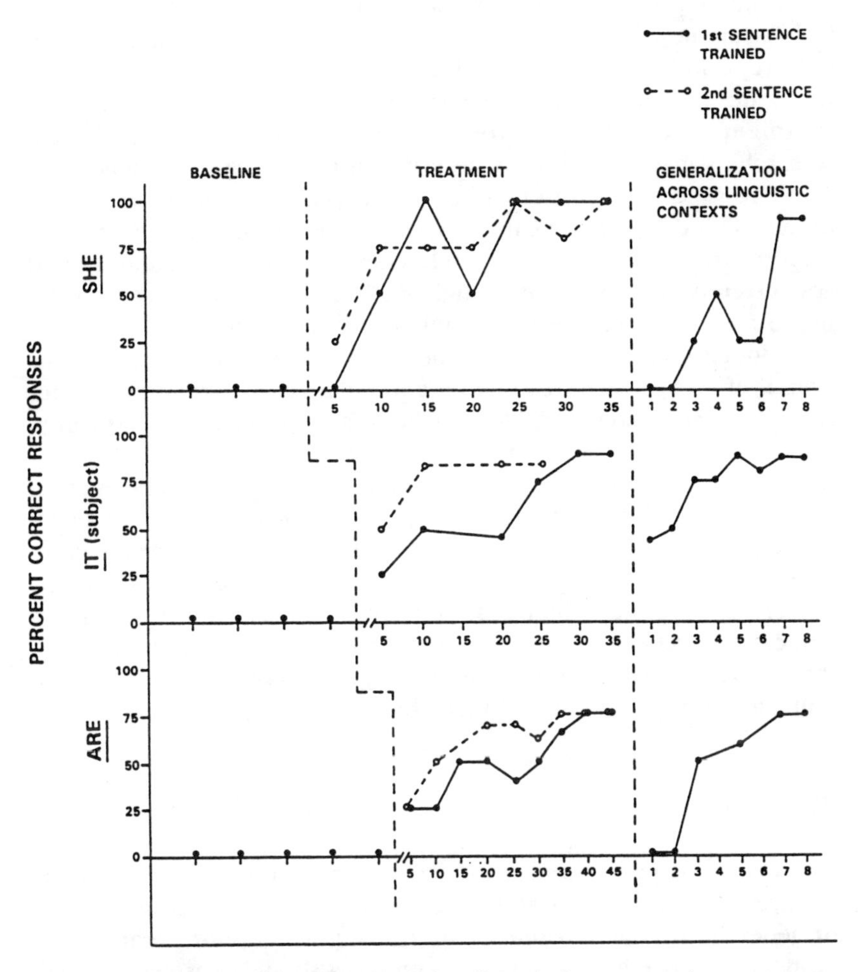

Figure 2–2. Examples of multiple-baseline design across three grammar targets. Structured probes were used for baseline and generalization assessments. For assessment of generalization across linguistic contexts, untrained visual stimuli that required the grammatical feature in untrained sentences were interspersed with stimuli used to evoke sentences during training.

generalization and maintenance measures collected in a nontreatment setting. When training reversed the behavior and initiations decreased in the treatment setting, unobtrusive generalization probes in the nontreatment setting indicated that initiations decreased in that setting also. When initiations were reinstated in treatment, they increased again in the nontreatment setting. Maintenance probes indicated that initiations remained high in the treatment setting but were decreasing in the nontreatment setting.

A major problem with withdrawal and reversal designs is that clinical researchers may object to reversing a client's performance for even a short period to establish experimental control. Thus, even though A-B-A-B designs are considered more powerful in demonstrating experimental control than are multiple-baseline designs, clinical researchers may often opt for use of multiple-baseline designs.

The last design to be described briefly is the alternating treatments design. This design may be used to determine which of two treatments is more effective for changing a behavior. Treatments are administered concurrently, usually within a single session or day, and counterbalancing to control order effects is required. Generalization measures may be included as part of the measurement of treatment effectiveness. However, if effects of each treatment are to be kept separate, different but related target behaviors must be treated (and counterbalanced across subjects) during the alternating treatments phase.

In the past, within-subject experimental research has been more common in clinical psychology and special education than in speech-language pathology. Indeed, some of the studies of language intervention described in subsequent chapters were probably conducted not by speech-language pathologists but by psychologists. However, as more clinical researchers discover the power and elegance of these designs, their use in investigating treatment and generalization effects in communication disorders should increase.

SUMMARY

Measuring generalization effects of treatment on language targets requires planning and considerable time and effort. Structured probes of generalization across one or more parameters must be arranged. Responses to trained and untrained exemplars should be assessed in new settings and with new listeners. Results of these structured probes of generalization can indicate the degree of generalization that is occurring during or after treatment.

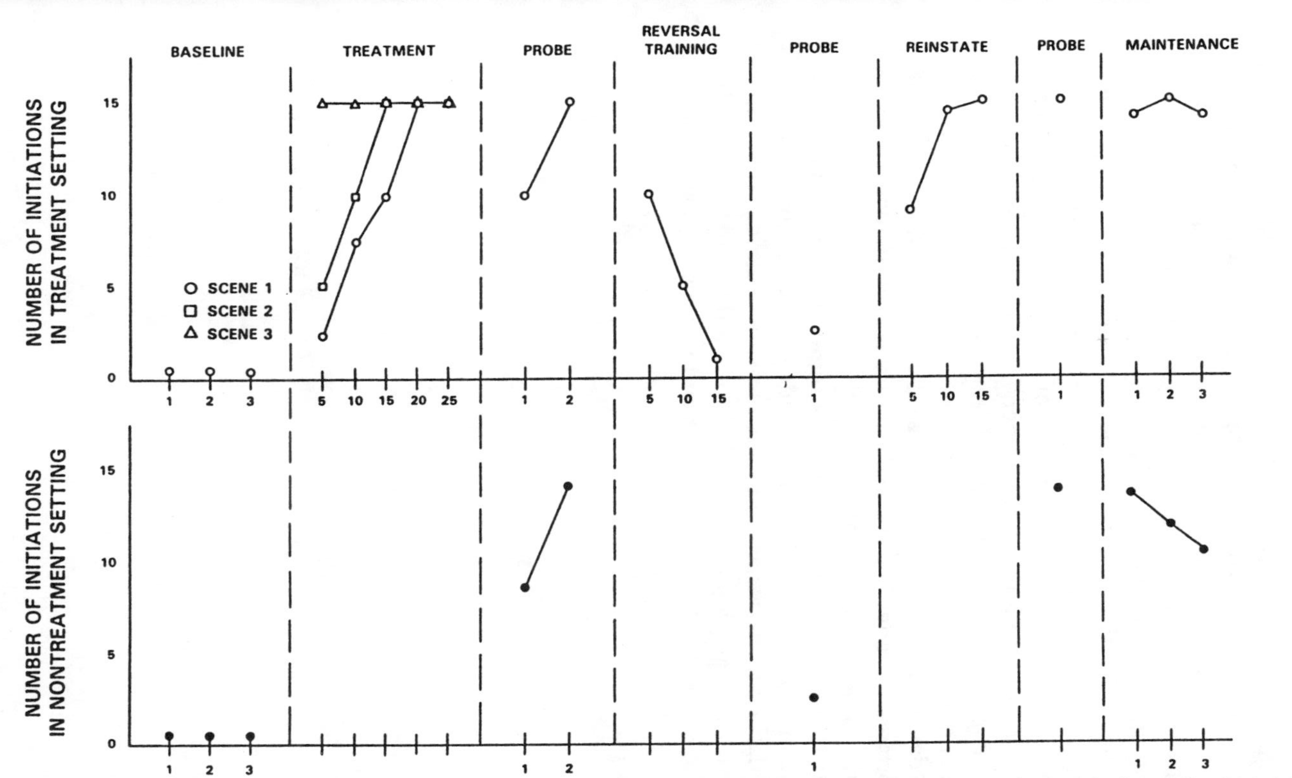

Figure 2–3. Example of an A-B-A-B reversal design with three maintenance measures. Treatment consisted of practice in initiating during role-playing of scenes requiring verbal initiations to request objects, activities, or help, with prompts and feedback. Generalization probes occurred in both treatment and nontreatment settings during 20-minute unobtrusive observations, during which 15 opportunities for initiations occurred. Data show generalization to nontreatment setting and some maintenance, although initiations in the nontreatment setting show a decline.

Probes of generalization to natural environments are considered the most rigorous tests of generalization. Results of generalization measures of spontaneous occurrence of the language target in natural environments is necessary to make informed decisions about termination of treatment on a target and about modifying the treatment program to promote generalization.

Although collection of accurate measures of generalization of language target behaviors may add yet another task to the responsibilities of the language clinician, such measures must become an integral part of the clinical intervention process. Generalization efforts may become a bridge between clinician and parents or caretakers, ensuring that these adults share in the language intervention process. Involving significant others in data collection should result in their increased awareness of the importance of language and communication in the daily interactions of the language-disordered child.

In the following chapters, the generalization measurement procedures used in numerous studies may provide practicing clinicians with ideas for data collection that are usable in many treatment situations. As these measures are described, think about modifications that might make them applicable to various clients and various language targets.

Chapter 3
Response Generalization

Recall that response generalization is observed to occur when language behaviors that are topographically similar to those trained are produced in response to similar stimuli, subsequent to training. These untrained responses have not been reinforced, and yet they occur as new responses based upon old learning. A nonbehaviorally oriented clinician may think of these instances as rule-generated productions; i.e., the child has detected a pattern among the trained responses and applies this rule to new instances that conform to the pattern detected.

From a behavioral point of view, response generalization may be thought of as generalization across behaviors, usually behaviors that somehow resemble the target behaviors. For example, the application of contingencies to increase the frequency of correct production of plural *-s* on a small set of nouns results in production of plural *-s* on numerous untrained nouns. Response generalization may co-occur with stimulus generalization, for example, in nontraining settings or with nontraining listeners.

The term *response generalization* has also been applied when changes occur in behaviors that are *not* similar to those under treatment, a broader definition of response generalization than one limited to changes in untreated behaviors that are topographically similar to the target behavior. Under this definition, response generalization is observed to occur when one behavior is systematically altered and other behaviors that have not been targets of intervention also change. For example, several investigators of generalization in autistic children have observed that self-stimulatory behaviors decrease when language behaviors increase (see Chapter 5). As another example, a nonverbal child who routinely showed aggression against adults in order to avoid certain situations was taught a manual gesture for "Let me out." As a result, aggression decreased, even though no contingencies were applied to it (Carr, Newsom, and Binkoff, 1980). Since any similarities that may have existed between self-stimulation and language or between aggression and a manual gesture are not readily apparent, perhaps the term *response generalization* is not suitable to describe such co-occurring changes. For purposes of this chapter, changes in such dissimilar behaviors will not be considered.

HOW SIMILAR IS SIMILAR?

The determination of whether a behavior is the same or different from that targeted for change depends on the definition of the target behavior (Drabman, Hammer, and Rosenbaum, 1979). Suppose the target is narrowly defined, e.g., *is* production in simple declarative sentences of the type "This is a (label)." If subsequent production of sentences such as "My mom is in the kitchen" or "That dog is fighting" or "Is that mine?" were correctly produced, these would be examples of response generalization across linguistic contexts. If, however, the target is broadly defined as *is* production in all sentences, then the other examples would not be considered response generalization, but merely successful behavior change, according to the definition of Drabman and associates. Such a definition, of course, begs the question of just how the desired response should be defined.

The problem of defining the boundaries of a desired response so that some degree of response generalization can be measured goes back a number of years. Skinner addressed it in 1953 when he reported that researchers tend to divide behavior into separate behavioral acts or units and then try to explain *response generalization, transfer*, or *response induction* in terms of responses that possess identical elements. In contrast to this approach, Skinner (1953) cautioned against dividing behavior into hard and fast units (responses), stressing instead the ultimately continuous nature of behavior (pp. 93–94). A more useful way of explaining transfer is to say that the elements, or "behavioral atoms," that are part of responses are strengthened whenever responses containing those elements are reinforced (Skinner, 1953). Verbal behavior supplies many good examples of such elements or behavioral atoms. Thus, when desired language responses are consequated in such a way as to increase their probability of occurrence, the component atoms, whether they are speech sounds or morphemes, are also strengthened.

FORMATION OF RESPONSE CLASSES

Untrained behaviors that change as a result of training on a few discrete behaviors have been described as members of the same *response class* (Guess, Keogh, and Sailor, 1978). If a controlled experiment showed that training on simple IS sentences resulted in increased correct production of both simple and transformed sentences, then we can conclude that the IS sentences were all members of the same response class. Of course, correct production of all IS sentences must have been equally low in frequency before treatment began. While the membership of response classes may be predicted by linguistic analysis, the formation of a response class can only be determined empirically, by controlled experimental analysis. Indeed, there is some evidence that grammatical categories that are distinct linguistically, such as subject and object noun phrases or copular and auxiliary forms of *is* and *are*, may not belong to separate response classes (Hegde, 1980; Hegde and McConn, 1981; McReynolds and Engmann, 1974).

GENERALIZATION ACROSS BEHAVIORS

While the various definitions of response generalization can be confusing, the following sections serve to illustrate what may be termed response generalization, at least by some researchers. The untrained responses measured bear some resemblance to the responses trained within therapy and were shown to have changed (increased in frequency) subsequent to training. Therefore, we can conclude that a response class was formed, which included the trained and untrained responses. The resemblance among the responses can be thought of as similarities within the linguistic domains of grammar (morphology and syntax), early semantic relational meanings, or referential meanings (word label for referent). Thus, based on our knowledge of language, we anticipate correct production of certain untrained morpheme combinations, sentences, or labels after training on a small subset of those morphemes or sentences. This is what we may think of as rule-learning.

Intraverbal Generalization

As an alternative to the term *response generalization across linguistic contexts*, Hegde (1985) proposed the term *intraverbal generalization*. For the most part, grammatical language targets require both a change in the stimulus and the response to be appropriate. For example, we wouldn't want untrained sentences such as "She is swimming" to occur in response to training stimuli such as a picture of a boy running and a request to tell about the picture. We seek generalization of the *is* and *–ing* portions of the response, combined with novel sentence subjects and verbs. Thus, both stimulus and response generalization are required for successful grammar learning, and the term *intraverbal generalization* captures this generalization across linguistic contexts. Hegde (1985) further describes *substitution* responses and *expansion* responses. When novel content words, such as nouns and verbs, are substituted for the trained content words while the grammatical function words remain constant, we have substitution responses. In the previous *is* + *-ing* examples, substitution responses might include sentences such as "The ice is melting" and "A duck is flying" after training on examples that did not contain these content words. Expansion responses are sentences that include the trained grammatical feature, but within longer or rearranged sentences. For example, after possessive or plural morphemes are trained, these grammatical morphemes are produced within various sentence positions, e.g., "Grandma's house is in the country," "I like Mother's cookies," "She bought games, marbles, and party hats," and "Prizes were given to the winners."

When or if intraverbal generalization occurs, language treatment becomes more efficient. Training on a small number of examples should result in many novel productions that include the target grammatical morpheme.

In the late 1960's and early 1970's research on language training appeared from two major groups. West Coast researchers studied the effects of programmed conditioning, primarily with dysphasic, nonlanguage children, using group research designs. The Monterey Language Program (Gray and Ryan, 1973), a program of 40 individualized language training units for which users must be certified, was a result of this research. Another group of researchers, based in Kansas, was studying the effects of operant conditioning on mentally retarded individuals, using single-subject research designs. In the following sections these studies will be reviewed as they offer data on response generalization across linguistic contexts, or intraverbal generalization.

The Monterey Program

Research on early attempts to develop a programmed conditioning procedure for use with language-impaired children defined response generalization rather broadly, requiring that production of targets in *spontaneous* language be part of the definition. These researchers attempted to develop a programmed conditioning method "whereby the child gains the facility to spontaneously generate correct and appropriate constructions within a given corpus of content and function words, i.e., response generalization." (Gray and Fygetakis, 1968). While pre- and post-treatment spontaneous language samples were used to assess target generalization, setting and listeners for these samples were not always specified. In some cases, 2- to 3-minute samples were recorded during Show and Tell time in the classroom, with teachers asking questions. The authors stressed that children freely constructed their own sentences with no prompting, often self-correcting when targets were incorrect (Fygetakis and Gray, 1970). Grammatical targets, such as copular and auxiliary *is*, interrogative *is*, *the*, adjectives, prepositions, and *wh-* questions were trained in a sequence of steps, and targets were subsequently produced in spontaneous samples, reportedly 7 to 18 weeks later. These authors proposed that response generalization occurs at two levels. At one level, target responses generalize to different but appropriate language situations, and at the other level, responses are incorporated into new linguistic constructions that are correct and appropriate. The programmed conditioning created an environment wherein the child's language system could process linguistic input designed to present little ambiguity or confusion, permitting the child to correctly identify rules of language. Conditioning attention to linguistic structure could activate the child's abilities to formulate linguistic rules (Fygetakis and Ingram, 1973). Thus, the Monterey Language Program that grew out of the work by these authors was influenced by both behavioral and psycholinguistic theories.

Early Generative Responding Studies

In contrast to the program developed by Gray, Ryan, and Fygetakis, research on language learning in mentally retarded individuals was solely operant in nature. In the early 1970's a number of operant studies showed that programming consequences to change a small set of language behaviors resulted in generalized responses to untrained exemplars. Language behaviors such as production of bound morphemes, present-progressive sentences, *wh-* questions, and verb inflections were trained by use of imitation, modeling, prompting, shaping, chaining, fading, and reinforcement. Measures of generalization were usually highly structured, occurred in the treatment setting, and were carried out by the trainer; only untrained picture or object stimuli were used to evoke the learned response within new linguistic environments. This recombining of learned elements of the language system into novel recombinations to describe newly encountered events has been termed "generative responding." Since these early studies did not report whether or not such generative responding also occurred when appropriate in the subject's natural environment (as spontaneous language sampling could have shown), it may be assumed that such measurement did not occur. If such generalization did occur, it could be called "recombinatory generalization" (Rogers-Warren and Warren, 1981), and it is this kind of generalization of course, that is the goal of a comprehensive language intervention program.

A brief summary of some of the early generative responding studies, mainly within-subject designs, will illustrate the range of language structures that were targets and the kinds of response generalization that occurred. A review and analysis of generative responding studies that sought to teach grammar to mentally retarded children can also be found in Welch (1981). Keep in mind that these targets were not chosen because they were developmentally appropriate for the client, nor was much attention paid to functionality of the language behaviors, although this became a concern in later investigations. Table 3–1 summarizes these studies and provides pertinent details for each.

Bound morphemes that were trained by operant techniques included plural allomorphs (Guess, Sailor, Rutherford, and Baer, 1968; Sailor, 1971), past-tense morphemes (Clark and Sherman, 1975; Schumaker and Sherman, 1970), progressive morpheme with auxiliary (Lutzker and Sherman, 1974; Schumaker and Sherman, 1970), participles (Clark and Sherman, 1975), and possessive allomorphs (Hegde, Noll, and Pecora, 1979). These trained responses generalized to untrained items in response to verbal stimuli used in training, usually *wh-* questions and some cloze sentence frames.

Present progressive sentences [N + *is* + V + *ing*] were trained in language-impaired (Wheeler and Sulzer, 1970), hearing-impaired (Bennett and Ling, 1972), and mentally retarded children (Lutzker and Sherman, 1974). Sometimes the contrast between singular *is* and plural *are* was trained (Garcia, Guess, and Byrnes, 1973; Lutzker and Sherman, 1974). In these studies, as in the studies of bound morphemes, the trained responses generalized to untrained exemplars in response to the verbal antecedents used in training. *Wh-* questions, such as "What color?," were trained by Twardosz and Baer (1973) to occur not in response to verbal stimuli but to visual presentation of a card. Color and size adjectives within noun phrases were trained by Martin (1975), and generalization to untrained items within two nontreatment settings and to two nontraining adults was observed.

Although subjects for many of the aforementioned studies were retarded individuals, operant research was also carried out with nonretarded children. Sentences with third-person pronouns were trained in language-impaired children, with resulting generalization to untrained exemplars in response to the verbal stimuli used in training, both in the clinical setting (Hegde and Gierut, 1979) and at home with mothers presenting the stimuli (Hegde, Noll, and Pecora, 1979).

Pronouns and self-referent speech were trained in mentally retarded children by Rubin and Stolz (1974), who found pronoun production in

Table 3–1. Operant Generative Responding Studies of Language Training

Authors	Subjects	Language Target	Generalization
Guess, Sailor, Rutherford, and Baer (1968)	1 MR child	Noun + plural *-s/-z*	To untrained objects in response to "What do you see?" used in training.
Clark and Sherman (1975)	3 MR adolescents and 4 disadvantaged children	Past and future tense and verb participle	To untrained items in response to verbal stimuli used in training.
Lutzker and Sherman (1974)	3 MR subjects and 2 normal subjects	Subject-verb agreement: [Noun + (s) + *is/are* + verb + *-ing*	To untrained sentences in response to "What's happening?" used in training.
Hegde, Noll, and Pecora (1979)	2 language-delayed children	Pronouns [*he, she, it*], auxiliary and copular [*'s, was*], and possessive [*'s, -s/-z*]	To untrained items, untrained linguistic contexts, and untrained items with mother at home, in response to verbal stimuli used in training.
Wheeler and Sulzer (1970)	1 speech-deficient child	Complete sentences: [Noun + *is* + verb + *-ing*]	To untrained items in response to "What do you see?" used in training.
Bennett and Ling (1972)	1 hearing-impaired child	Complete sentences: [*The* noun + *is* + verb + *-ing*]	To untrained items in response to "Tell me about this" used in training.
Garcia, Guess, and Byrnes (1973)	1 MR child	Singular and plural sentences: "That is one ________" and "These are two ________."	To untrained items in response to visual stimuli only, no model to imitate as in training.
Twardosz and Baer (1973)	2 MR adolescents	*wh-* questions: "What [color, letter, number]?"	To untrained items in response to presentation of a card.
Martin (1975)	2 MR children	Color and size adjectives: [adjective + noun]	To untrained items in response to "What is this?" and to nontraining setting and persons.
Hegde and Gierut (1979)	1 language-delayed child	Subject and object pronouns and auxiliary *are*: *She* reads. Dog bites *him*. Cars *are* stopping.	To untrained sentences in response to verbal stimuli used in training.
Rubin and Stolz (1974)	1 MR adolescent	Pronouns and self-referent speech: [*I, my, you, your, she, he*] + noun	To untrained combinations in response to teacher's *wh-* questions in classroom, with extended training.

untrained combinations in response to teacher questions in the classroom after training was instituted within the classroom. In addition, a decrease in idiosyncratic speech was noted. Training autistic children in production of simple sentences and then compound sentences conjoined with *and* resulted in generalization to novel simple and compound sentences in response to pictures (Stevens-Long and Rasmussen, 1974; Stevens-Long, Schwarz, and Bliss, 1976). Anecdotal teacher reports of spontaneous use of compound sentences within the classroom were also noted.

The preceding language targets were brief units, such as morphemes, phrases, and sentences. Operant procedures were also applied to more ambitious language units, such as multi-sentence conversational sequences. Garcia (1974) trained a five-turn conversational speech sequence, which consisted of presentation of a picture, to which the child responded "What is that?", an answer by the trainer ("This is a ________. What do you see?"), to which the child replied "It's a ________," and finally the question "Do you want the ________?" and the response "Yes, I do." Although the two subjects learned these responses to untrained pictures, little generalization to two other people in different settings was evident until probe pictures were intermixed with training pictures reinforced on a VR 3 schedule. This "conversational" sequence seems quite artificial and contrived, especially when viewed from the current emphasis on pragmatics. Still, this was an early attempt to program language beyond the sentence unit.

Another attempt to train more complex verbal behaviors by operant procedures was carried out by Keilitz, Tucker, and Horner (1973), who trained three retarded adolescents to respond to directives ("Tell me what you saw on the news") and questions ("What else did you see on the news today?") about television news presentations. Since each news program contained different events, response generalization (as well as stimulus generalization) could be observed in the language produced. Results indicated increases in the percentage of accurate verbal responses over baseline measures. When each news item was viewed separately and then was followed by opportunities to respond, verbal statements were more accurate than when the entire program was viewed prior to response opportunities.

Taken together, these studies provide a sample of language training procedures that have resulting in various kinds of response, or intraverbal, generalization. However, generalization to spontaneous production in natural environments was not measured in these studies, and it seems unlikely that such generalization would have occurred. Results of such operant research led to an optimistic view that "...an operant technology presently exists for the establishment and maintenance of expressive speech..." (Garcia and DeHaven, 1974, p. 176) and the prediction that language training technology would eventually establish normal speech.

TYPE OF LANGUAGE TARGETS: SOME COMPARISONS

When the language target consists of two or more word utterances, syntactic rules for word order must be taught. Training is done on one or a few combinations, and intraverbal generalization to similar combinations is assessed. The goal is to teach the underlying rule (e.g., [noun + verb] or [agent + action]), rather than the surface form (e.g., "doggie eat"). The words in the child's vocabulary must include a sufficient number of nouns (agents) and verbs (actions) so that training can use some but not all of them, leaving some untrained vocabulary with which to test for generalization to untrained exemplars. Structured probes may be constructed to elicit various combinations, such as [Trained Noun + Untrained Verb], [Untrained Noun + Trained Verb], and [Untrained Noun + Untrained Verb]. Thus, generalization patterns on structured probes may be systematically measured. In analyzing generalization data, it would be important to include a breakdown of combination types, so that teaching strategies could be altered if certain patterns were not being generalized. In addition to intraverbal generalization as measured by structured probes, measures of spontaneous conversational speech are needed to assess generalization to spontaneously produced language in natural environments.

Some syntactic classes do not contain many possible exemplars (pronouns, for example), whereas other classes may contain a very large number (nouns, for example). Thus, some syntactic strings may be taught, which include *some* words that rarely change and one word that often changes. For instance, requests such as "I want ________" or "Give me ________" include two words that seldom vary (as long as intent remains the same) and one word that will vary depending on the item desired. A question arises here as to just how much change should be required in order to constitute evidence of generalization. A stringent criterion would require that multiple examples from each word class must be produced before the resulting behavior is called "generalization." Using the previous example, we'd want to hear "You like apple" and "They hate peas" as well as "I want cookie" before we would say a child has a syntactic rule for [Pronoun + State-verb + Noun]. In addition, we'd want to know whether such utterances were prompted with a *wh-* question such as "What do you want?" or were uttered without verbal prompting, in appropriate, nontherapy situations, before we would agree that the child is showing the desired generalized language behavior.

Results of generalization subsequent to syntax training have been disappointing when more stringent criteria for generalization are applied (Warren et al., 1980). After training on 12 syntactic forms via the Guess, Sailor, and Baer program, four retarded subjects showed a mean of four forms generalized to the natural environment (33 per cent) over approximately seven months. After similar training on 23 forms, four language-delayed (nonretarded) preschool children showed a mean of five forms generalized (22 per cent). The investigators concluded that changes in the forms chosen for training and the manner in which they were trained might have achieved greater generalization.

Even though little syntactic generalization occurred, when the same data were analyzed for semantic relations expressed and for communicative function of the utterance, greater generalization to the natural environment was noted (Warren et al., 1980). For two mildly delayed children who had been trained with multiple exemplars of each semantic relationship, strong generalization effects for five of the seven semantic relations were shown. However, the one severely retarded child displayed no syntactic or semantic generalization. When generalization of pragmatic functions of language was examined, some success was also observed. Concurrent with training on nine different exemplars of the control pragmatic function (e.g., "I want" or "Give me") a strong acceleration in use of control utterances, regardless of form, was demonstrated for one child. This child used *untrained* syntactic forms to control the environment. Again, the retarded child did not show any increase in the control function outside of therapy as a result of training.

The data reported by Warren and colleagues (1980) suggest that generalization of correct syntax is a more difficult skill than is generalization of semantic or pragmatic skills. The greater generalization across semantic relations suggests that early language-rule learning occurs across semantic, not syntactic, categories—a phenomenon found in normally developing children acquiring their first language. The successful generalization of the control function of language, expressed with various exemplars, also parallels the development of communicative functions in normal children, e.g., the proto-imperatives described by Bates, Camaioni, and Volterra (1975). It may be that selection of early language goals based on the results of developmental research on the normal population would result in more successful training of language within disordered populations. What is needed is systematic research to determine the conditions of generalization failure and generalization success. Only such controlled research can reveal more efficient and less efficient sequences of language training (Brinker and Bricker, 1979).

RESPONSE GENERALIZATION IN MODELING STUDIES

One of several approaches to language training is modeling, a procedure based on observational learning theory as applied by Bandura and Harris (1966). A number of studies have employed a modeling approach for teaching various language target behaviors in various populations (Carroll, Rosenthal, and Brysh, 1972; Courtright and Courtright, 1976 and 1979; Haynes and Haynes, 1980; Leonard, 1975; Prelock and Panagos, 1980; Wilcox and Leonard, 1978). For the modeling approach, the child is not asked to produce immediate imitations of a model, but to listen carefully to a series of models because it will soon be the child's turn to speak. Sometimes the person modeling produces a percentage of incorrect responses, which are not reinforced. By observing which of the model's productions are reinforced, the child problem-solves to derive a rule for correct productions. If the model and the child are given identical visual stimuli for target productions, this is called *imitative modeling*; if the child is given a similar but not identical set of stimuli, this is called *nonimitative modeling*.

In a study designed to investigate patterns of generalization to untrained examples, Wilcox and Leonard (1978) trained three *wh-* question words (*what, where,* and *who*) and two auxiliaries (*is* and *does*) by modeling procedures to 24 language-impaired children. After each experimental group reached criterion on one sentence (e.g., *what* + *is*), generalization to untrained combinations of *wh-* question words and auxiliaries was assessed, using pictures and verbal antecedents such as, "Ask me what the boy is catching." Results revealed that once subjects learned a specific auxiliary transposition in a trained form, it was generalized to other *wh-* questions requiring it. Neither *is*-training alone nor *does*-training alone, however, resulted in generalization to the other auxiliary form. This suggests that each auxiliary morpheme was a separate response class. More generalization was observed after training on *is* sentences than on *does* sentences. Subjects trained on *where* showed more generalization to untrained *wh-* questions than those trained on *who* and *what*. Clinical implications of these results may guide clinicians in choosing language targets with the greatest potential for generalization, i.e., *where* questions and *is* auxiliaries.

In terms of response generalization, this study provides some interesting patterns of recombinations of trained forms with untrained forms. Evidently, some transfer of learning was occurring, but it was not systematic across all language forms. Since this study did not include a measure of the use of trained forms in either trained or novel combinations within spontaneously produced conversational speech, it is unknown whether or not spontaneous generalization to the natural environment occurred.

An intervention study using a modeling approach that did include measurement of pre-treatment and post-treatment spontaneous usage of the language target was reported by Prelock and Panagos (1980). The language target for the mentally retarded subjects was agent-agent-object constructions, and all three words were required for correct responses. After five training sessions over 3 weeks, statistical analysis revealed significant improvement for both mimicry (immediate imitation) and modeling groups but no significant differences in the number of correct responses produced under each condition. However, structured generalization probes with novel pictures showed that the modeling subjects performed better than mimicry subjects on both mimicry and modeling generalization tasks. Spontaneous usage of the language target in a free-play setting was significantly greater for the modeling subjects than for the mimicry subjects. Prelock and Panagos concluded that the imitative modeling approach was more effective than the mimicry approach across linguistic, cognitive, and conversational domains of learning.

This study provides a good example of the use of two levels of measurement of generalization—response generalization to untrained examples (novel pictures) and generalization to spontaneous production in a natural environment. When both measures are included in the experimental design, patterns of generalization across two dimensions of generalization can be observed.

As the results of these two modeling studies indicate, modeling procedures have resulted in some successful achievement of response (intraverbal) generalization. After training on some examples of the language target, correct similar responses were produced for novel, untrained examples. In addition, subjects in the Prelock and Panagos study also showed generalization to spontaneous production in a nontreatment setting.

CROSS-MODAL GENERALIZATION: COMPREHENSION AND PRODUCTION

A number of studies have investigated response generalization across receptive and expressive language modalities, asking questions such as, "Does training to increase comprehension of language targets affect production of those targets?" and, conversely, "Does training on production of language targets result in comprehension of those targets?" Research using normal children and nonsense words or words or letters in a foreign language have shown some transfer across modalities, with production training showing greater cross-modal response generalization than comprehension training (Connell and McReynolds, 1981; Cromer and Ault, 1979).

Studies training language-disordered children in comprehension or production of language targets, or both, have produced discrepant results. An early study by Guess (1969) trained plurals in comprehension alone and in production alone, and results indicated little reciprocal generalization in the two retarded children. Similarly, little comprehension to production transfer was shown in other training studies (Guess and Baer, 1973; Miller, Cuvo, and Borakove, 1977; Ruder, Smith, and Hermann, 1974). However, other studies (Cuvo and Riva, 1980; Keller and Bucher, 1979; Paluszek and Feintuch, 1979; Ruder, Hermann, and Schiefelbusch, 1977) have reported considerable cross-modal transfer. Apparently, cross-modal response generalization varies widely among subjects and may be affected by numerous factors.

Several factors that may affect cross-modal generalization were explored in a study of retarded and normal children by Bucher and Keller (1981). Children were trained to identify pictures when given verbal labels and then were tested for production of the labels. Results showed that transfer was affected by stimulus factors (familiarity of the pictures), response factors (length or similarity of nonsense labels), context factors (intermixed comprehension and production trials), and training factors (repeated testing). Similar patterns of transfer were observed for normal and retarded children.

Most of these studies of cross-modal transfer have used nonsense or foreign-language nouns to label figures or objects as the language target. Some used a bound plural morpheme (Guess and Baer, 1973; Holdgrafer and McReynolds, 1975; Paluszek and Feintuch, 1979). None reported any observation of generalization of trained behaviors to natural environments; indeed, when nonsense forms were trained, such generalization would not be desired. Nevertheless, the studies of cross-modal response generalization were designed to explore issues in lexical acquisition and morphological rule learning and are limited in scope to response generalization across receptive-expressive language behaviors. Studies of the effects of training on comprehension or production of language behaviors, which include measures of natural environment generalization (of both comprehension and production), are necessary if we are to assess the relative benefits of separate training in the two modalities for clinical language intervention.

MATRIX TRAINING STUDIES

A number of studies of the generalization of trained language responses to untrained language behaviors or new combinations of trained language behaviors have used a matrix training approach (Karlan, Brenn-White, Lentz, Hodur, Egger, and Frankoff, 1982; Romski and Ruder, 1984; Striefel, Wetherby, and Karlan, 1976 and 1978). In these studies, a matrix or grid is designed, with one set of language components (e.g., nouns) along the ordinate and another set of language components (e.g., verbs) along the abscissa. After a subset of two-word combinations is trained, the remaining untrained combinations can be assessed to determine whether a rule has been generalized. Trained items can be those along the matrix borders or those on a diagonal. Results of these studies have demonstrated the development of "rule-bound" behavior, since matrix training apparently resulted in an ability to recognize that events in the environment had distinct components (actions, objects, or descriptive characteristics) and that each component was represented by a unique linguistic element (verb, noun, or adjective) that could be combined in rule-governed ways.

This matrix training approach was applied by Karlan and colleagues (1982) to teach four impaired children functioning at a language age of approximately two years to manually sign verb-noun phrases. Training sessions were carried out once or twice daily by a teacher or clinician within a classroom where simultaneous communication was used throughout the day. The four students were paired, and up to 15 trials were presented to each student during each session. The 64-item pool of eight verbs (e.g., *pick up, carry, put*) and eight nouns (e.g., *cup, chair, crayon*) were actions and objects that occurred commonly in the classroom and that would be likely to be used in communicating, according to the classroom staff. A diagonal step-wise sequence of training items was followed, representing the potentially most efficient progression through the matrix (see Figure 3–1). This sequence introduced verb contrasts early in the sequence, thus eliminating a problem of verb learning that had been encountered in an earlier study (Striefel et al., 1976). Trials consisted of an action on an object performed by the adult or a peer, followed by the question, "What did I/he/she do?" Correct signs were consequated with both social praise and an edible reward; partially or totally incorrect signs were consequated with a "No," repetition of the question and action, and a model of the two-sign combination. Correct imitations of the model were reinforced. Incorrect imitations were consequated with "No" and physical guidance through the sign as the adult restated the verb-noun phrase. As items were learned, training sessions included three review trials of previously learned items randomly interspersed with new items. Criterion performance was 11 of the 12 nonreview items correct for three consecutive sessions.

After criterion was met on a subset of three training items, both training probes and generalization probes were conducted. Training

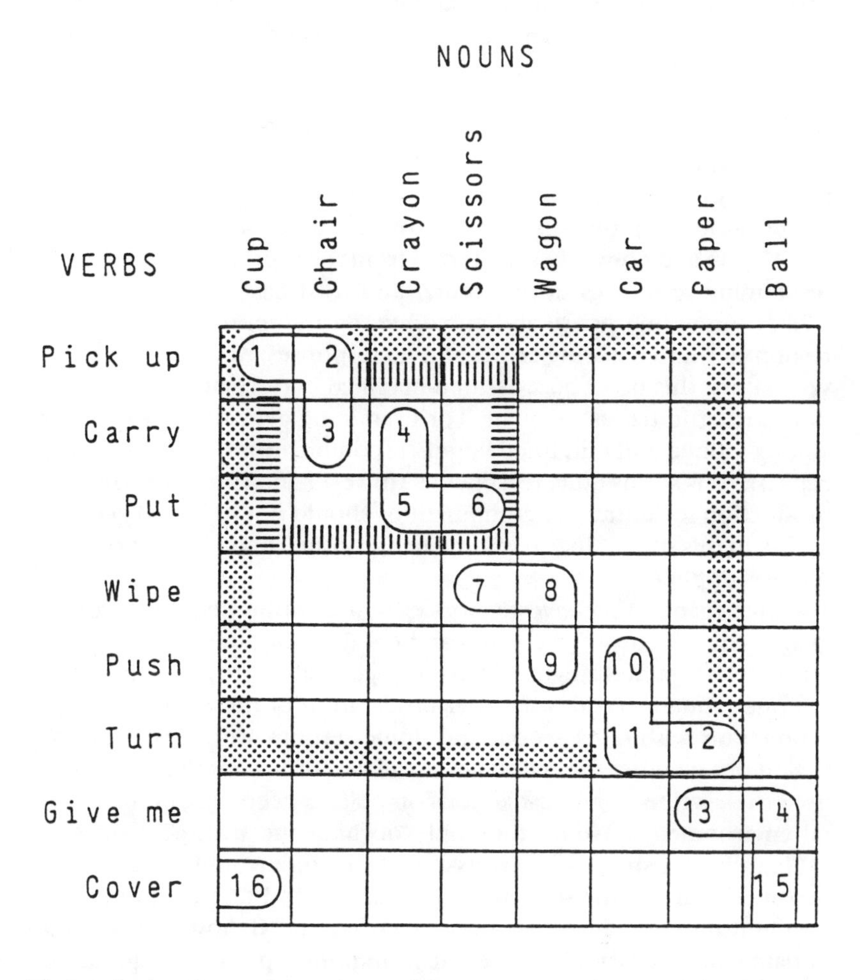

Figure 3–1. Expressive verb-noun training matrix. Numbered cells represent training items; circled items indicate training subsets. Remaining verb-noun combinations permit assessment of generalization to untrained verb-noun pairs. (From Karlan, G., Brenn-White, B., Lentz, A., Hodur, P., Egger, D., and Frankoff, D. (1982). Establishing generalized, productive verb-noun usage in a manual language system with moderately handicapped children. *Journal of Speech and Hearing Disorders. 47,* 33. Copyright 1982 by the American Speech-Language-Hearing Association. Reprinted by permission.)

probes included all novel recombinations of trained elements, and generalization probes included combinations of trained and not-yet-trained verbs and nouns. Results indicated that two of the students performed well on probes of trained and recombined elements and also showed a pattern of increasingly correct responding to combinations of trained verb–untrained noun. On the total 64-item probe, these two students moved from 0 per cent and 2 per cent correct on the initial baseline to 78 per cent and 92 per cent correct on the final baseline. One student, more vocal than the others, was dropped because of her confusion of signs and words. This student had been paired with the other student who showed less learning. Thus, the overlapped diagonal matrix strategy was successful in developing generalized signed expression of verb-noun combinations in two of the three students studied.

Karlan and co-workers departed from the typical procedure of not reinforcing responses during initial and final baseline measures and probes, providing praise and an edible reward contingent on correct responding and ignoring errors and no responses. According to the investigators, this procedure assured maximal performance and motivation during initial assessment. For examining generalization patterns among trained and untrained linguistic combinations on a rather artificial task, this seems quite reasonable. However, increases in correct sign production for untrained combinations should not be called *generalization* in this study, since reinforcement contingent on correct responding was applied.

Like many other investigators examining a limited aspect of language generalization, these researchers did not attempt to find out whether the trained language behaviors generalized to spontaneous use in nontreatment settings. Further observation of these children's sign production within classroom and home settings would be necessary to find out whether the trained or novel verb-noun combinations were used to describe or request actions on objects occurring in their natural environments. Would they only occur if the treatment question "What did I/he/she do?" were asked? If so, there would seem to be little functional use for such signing behavior, and one could question the clinical significance of such "generalization." If, however, the child initiated the signs without verbal prompting—perhaps requesting a teacher to "pick up crayon" when the crayon had rolled out of reach—then a much larger kind of generalization is apparent. While it is interesting to note that the diagonal step-wise arrangement is an efficient way to teach verb-noun combinations, unless such language behavior is used communicatively by the learner, only a small step toward our goal of increased communicative effectiveness has been taken.

Another matrix study was designed to investigate cross-modal generalization as well as generalization to untrained combinations. The effectiveness of two treatments, speech alone versus speech-plus-sign, was examined using ten Down's syndrome children ranging in age from 4 to 7 years (Romski and Ruder, 1984). Children were taught to comprehend seven action-object combinations, using either speech or speech-plus-sign stimulation. Generalization to nine untreated combinations was assessed after criterion was reached, and generalization to speech (not sign) production for all 16 combinations was also assessed. These generalization probes were conducted in both the treatment setting and in a classroom, to examine setting generalization as well.

Results indicated that in comprehension some generalization to untreated combinations occurred (an average of 3.1 of the 9 possible combinations) and that treated combinations were maintained in the generalization probes. Although subjects erred on approximately six of the nine untreated combinations, they generally got *either* the action or the object correct, thus indicating some learning, since all target words were unknown at the beginning of the study. In production, few correct responses were noted, and these occurred almost exclusively on the treated items. Again, some (about one quarter) of the error responses included *either* the correct action or object. For all generalization measures, there were minimal differences between the speech alone and the speech-plus-sign conditions. However, there were individual children for whom the speech-plus-sign condition was both particularly beneficial or detrimental.

This study illustrates nicely how initial learning can occur while generalization to new combinations or to another modality (production) fails to occur. Both kinds of generalization were incomplete, indicating that additional programming specifically designed to promote generalization would be needed. To effect generalization to untreated combinations, perhaps a few more examples would need to be taught. To achieve generalization from comprehension to production, perhaps some specific oral responses would be necessary. The matrix approach allows for easy checking of generalization to untreated combinations, and the assessment of production (after training in comprehension) can reveal whether cross-modal generalization is occurring. These intervention techniques may be useful tools for clinicians who want to apply efficient and systematic instruction for two-word utterances.

The action and object words chosen for this study may have been a factor in the low rates of generalization. In order to control for prior knowledge, the words chosen were not particularly frequent or functional in natural environments. Verbs included *cover, pound,* and *toss,* and nouns included *clip, magnet,* and *penguin*. If more functional words for familiar objects could have been chosen individually for each child, perhaps more generalization would have occurred.

The diagonal step-wise matrix training approach has also been applied to teach profoundly retarded adults to respond appropriately to action-object commands (McCuller and Salzberg, 1984). As in the Romski and Ruder study, it was necessary to choose action and object words (e.g., *switch, flip, gasket, bobbin*) that were unknown to the subjects, and this resulted in words that would not be particularly useful in natural environments. Physical prompts, verbal praise, and edible rewards were used in concurrent-training sessions for pairs of action-object instructions. After criterion was met on concurrent-training, random-sequence sessions were used. These combined review trials, new trials, and recombined instructions. A multiple-baseline design across response sets was used to assess three groups of generalization probes.

The number of trials needed to reach criterion varied from 2,295 to 5,537 for the three mentally retarded subjects. Despite these differences among the subjects on training efficiency, subjects showed similar patterns on recombined instructions. These results suggest that a matrix training approach may be useful in teaching receptive language targets to profoundly retarded adults. Given frequently occurring, familiar, and functional actions and objects, generalization across untrained combinations might be expected more rapidly than for the unfamiliar words used by McCuller and Salzberg. Additionally, some generalization to the natural environment would be more likely. Additional research is needed to investigate the effectiveness of the matrix approach for achieving generalization to natural environments.

RESPONSE GENERALIZATION AND INCIDENTAL TEACHING

One way of eliminating the gap between use of language targets in therapy and use of them outside therapy is to do the therapy out in the natural environments. The incidental teaching approach developed by Hart and Risley is an attempt to do just that, using a preschool classroom as a natural environment. By collection of language samples within the classroom, changes in language targets other than those directly taught can be noted. Thus, one of the few investigations of response generalization that examined spontaneous language samples for occurrence of both target and nontarget language behaviors was reported by Hart and Risley (1980). After realizing that language training under close stimulus control often failed to generalize to any marked extent into spontaneous language use in uncontrolled situations, these investigators rearranged the preschool environment so that the language trained under controlled conditions was both functional and necessary for children to gain access to reinforcers available in the natural preschool environment (Hart and Risley, 1980). Such natural reinforcers as teacher attention, materials, and activities were manipulated by teachers in the classroom within brief one-to-one interactions with individual children.

An earlier study had demonstrated the effectiveness of an incidental teaching approach for increasing production of compound sentence forms in disadvantaged preschool children (Hart and Risley, 1975). The approach had established a response class, language use, that was likely to be generalized by stimulus similarity across settings and occasions and to be reinforced in a wide variety of stimulus conditions. In an attempt to discover unprogrammed side effects of the experimental investigation of compound sentence production, the spontaneous language sample data were re-examined. Data from the children receiving incidental teaching were compared with data from children in a Head Start program and a university preschool, who had not received incidental teaching. During free-play periods, 15-minute speech samples were recorded verbatim by one of three observers over nine months. One to four samples per week were collected, depending on the setting. Two general classes of behavior were examined: language use (defined as the occurrence of a word or a sentence) and language elaboration (defined as the occurrence of a different word or a nonbasic sentence type). Thus, words and sentences were measures of the occurrence of a response class, i.e., language use. When all occurrences of the trained language behaviors (compound sentences of the trained type, e.g., "I want *X* so I can *Y*") had been excluded from the data, major increases in rates of language use were found for the experimental children. Increases in language elaboration—i.e., numbers of different words and complex sentences used—accompanied the increases in language use. Children whose language was comparable to that of their disadvantaged peers in the Head Start program at the beginning of the school year were comparable on language measures with advantaged children in the university preschool by the end of the year. The marked changes in rates of language use and elaboration, which generalized across contexts and people, occurred only in the experimental setting, where incidental teaching had been used.

The increases in rates of language use were attributed to generalization from incidental teaching; increases in elaboration, in turn, were attributed to the increased language use (Hart and Risley, 1980). Thus, the incidental teaching approach, which reinforced child-initiated talk, had a domino effect, resulting in more complex language as children initiated more talk in a wider variety of circumstances. Whether or not such an effect would hold with language-disordered children remains to be investigated.

SUMMARY

Response generalization across linguistic contexts was one of the first kinds of language generalization to be systematically investigated. Most of the early studies used structured probes presenting untrained exemplars to determine whether trained morphemes and syntax patterns had generalized to new language content required by the untrained exemplars. Such generative responding was considered evidence that the child had learned a linguistic rule. Research comparing response generalization for syntactic, semantic, and pragmatic targets indicated that language targets that function to control the environment, regardless of form, may generalize most readily to the natural environment.

Intervention based on modeling procedures has been successful at achieving response generalization, and this may be a procedure that lends itself readily to measuring response generalization. Sets of stimuli similar to those used in training may be set aside to probe generalization across language behaviors, after modeling procedures have resulted in rule-learning for the training set. In comparison to immediate imitation procedures (mimicry), the modeling procedures were better at achieving generalization, both response generalization and generalization to a natural environment, at least in some studies.

Matrix training studies have explored response generalization by systematically pairing trained and untrained language components. The study by Karlan and associates showed successful response generalization of sign combinations in two of the three language-disordered children studied. Use of a planned matrix of target words may make learning more efficient, whether children are learning signs or speech.

Finally, Hart and Risley's incidental teaching procedures resulted in generalization across behaviors not directly trained. Both language use and language elaboration increased in the disadvantaged children studied. More recent studies have applied a modified version of incidental teaching to autistic children (see McGee et al., 1983, in Chapter 5).

Response generalization, which may also be called intraverbal generalization, may be considered the essential evidence that language rule-learning has occurred. Intervention on grammatical elements must result in application of a *rule* for using those elements in constructing sentences. Thus, response generalization is a necessary part of any language intervention program that includes grammatical targets. There are also rules for combining semantic elements and for expressing pragmatic functions. Less research has been done on these language targets, but generalization of these kinds of responses may be problematic, too. If clinicians are to avoid teaching numerous separate examples of each semantic category or each pragmatic function, response generalization, as well as stimulus generalization, must occur.

Chapter 4
Choosing Language Targets and Antecedent Events

There is a close connection between the content of language targets and the antecedent events used in treatment programs. The language behaviors chosen as targets must be appropriate for the client's cognitive and linguistic developmental level and functional in the child's natural environments. By observing what kinds of antecedent events trigger opportunities to produce the language targets within natural environments, clinicians may be able to arrange for similar antecedent events to be used during establishment and generalization phases of treatment.

When these target language behaviors are selected, the antecedent events that are common stimuli for them in natural environments must be considered. Rather than selecting simply "object labels" as a target, the clinician needs to consider what antecedent events trigger object labels for speakers in natural environments. More specifically, we might ask what events present a need for object labels in this individual client's natural environments. Children often label novel, interesting, or unexpected objects in their environments upon seeing them. Uttering the label draws or directs the attention of a listening adult to the object for a comment or confirmation of the label. Thus, sight of the object in the right context may be an antecedent event for object label production. Occasionally, an adult may even supply a verbal antecedent for an object label, asking "What's this/that?" and indicating an object. For normally developing children, these deliberate requests for object labels occur mostly with very young children who are just learning to talk. The adult usually thinks that the child knows the object's name and is giving the child a chance to display that knowledge. The adult's request for information is not "sincere," in Grice's terms.

For older, language-disordered children, the request for an object's name may also represent a test of the child's vocabulary rather than a sincere desire for an unknown label. As such, it is likely to be uttered by a teacher or clinician in a school-like situation. If, however, the child encounters a "What's this?" question in a nonschool environment, it is likely to be a sincere request for information. Perhaps the clinician who chooses to work on object labels needs to consider both types of "What's this?" questions. By choosing to teach labels for things that the child can identify but that others do *not* know, we can prepare the child for sincere requests for information that may occur within the natural environment. For example, a child's drawing may be used, with "What's this?" questions directed toward different objects drawn.

As the previous example of object labels taught to provide answers to anticipated requests for such labels illustrates, the content of the language target and the antecedent events that precede production of that target must match. When choosing language targets with a good potential for generalization, the clinician must simultaneously choose a variety of appropriate, naturally occurring antecedent events for teaching those targets. Such antecedent events may be either verbal or nonverbal. In the following sections, literature that has addressed the variables of language target content and antecedent events for language targets will be summarized, and conclusions concerning the relevance of these variables for achieving generalization will be drawn.

VERBAL ANTECEDENTS

One of the most interesting aspects of normal conversational language is its predictability, given knowledge of the context. While it is true that any speaker can produce novel utterances whenever there is a chance to say something, the rules dictating relevance to the topic at hand usually constrain the actual sentences uttered. Given knowledge of the context (e.g., setting, time, relationship of the speakers, and purposes for talking), we can often predict quite accurately what will be said.

As descriptive research on the pragmatic aspects of normal language is done, clinicians will learn more about the characteristics of normal language interactions and will be able to make better choices of verbal antecedents to use in language teaching. Consider some typical verbal antecedents used to elicit noun labels or present-progressive verbs, e.g., "What's this?" or "What's he doing?" Unless the asker truly doesn't know the answer, these violate the sincerity rule of conversational language. When asked by clinicians, they are obviously test questions, since the asker knows the answer and wants to find out if the child knows it or perhaps wants to give the child a chance to practice the language target. Although it may be argued that children will encounter test questions in school and thus need practice in supplying grammatically and semantically correct answers, we must remember that in conversations there are many and varied verbal antecedents for most language targets. Rarely is language use controlled by only one stimulus, even such a clear one as "What's this?" In the terms of behaviorists, "...any discriminative stimulus functions always and only in the right context ... in the wrong context, it doesn't function" (D. M. Baer, personal communication, July 28, 1984).

If our goal is only to get the child to produce object labels in response to test questions, we may be safe in using only "What's this?" as the verbal antecedent. However, our goal is much broader than this, so we need to plan for and provide a variety of verbal antecedents in teaching language targets if we are planning for generalization.

Use of Trained Verbal Antecedents

Generalization across verbal antecedents is one of the least investigated kinds of language generalization. When structured probes of generalization across settings and persons are used to measure generalization, the same verbal antecedents used in treatment are used to elicit the target language under the generalization conditions. One of the obvious reasons for this is that language targets are quite often only appropriate in response to the right verbal antecedent. For example, a client who is taught to name objects using "This is a ________" should not produce this sentence in response to *any* verbal antecedent but only in response to a limited few, such as "What's this?" or "Do you know what this is?" One could think of other situations, such as presenting a demonstration or lecture describing a number of objects, where no verbal antecedent precedes the sentence and where the object itself is the antecedent. Nevertheless, language targets such as "This is a ________" would be inappropriate responses to many verbal and nonverbal stimuli. Thus, when the clinician wants to assess generalization and needs many occurrences of the target, reliable elicitation devices are needed. Often, the easiest one to think of is the verbal antecedent used during therapy. However, this may not provide a good test of generalization, since the verbal antecedent may serve to trigger correct production.

As discussed in Chapter 2, it is often desirable to arrange for many opportunities for the target to occur when assessing generalization in order to avoid misleading percentages of correct responses, such as 50 per cent, based on one out of two opportunities. Therefore, in collecting generalization data, we are tempted to use a specific verbal antecedent that has a high probability of eliciting the language target. Consider the general directives used to elicit language in spontaneous language samples, "Tell me about ________" or "Tell me what's happening in these pictures" and the all-purpose questions to elicit progressive verb tense ("What's happening here?") or requests ("What do you want?"). These are often used in the final step of a teaching program, then may also be used for a structured probe of generalization to untrained examples, or to new persons, or in new settings. New pictures or objects may be used to check for response generalization, but the same verbal antecedents used in training are used to collect generalization data.

Many of the studies described in Chapters 5 and 6 on generalization across settings and persons used the same verbal antecedent spoken in training. If the verbal antecedent were the controlling stimulus, generalization across settings and persons might be readily demonstrated, but generalization to spontaneous production in natural environments, where a variety of verbal antecedents occur, would not be observed. Thus, generalization across verbal antecedents would not have been measured.

For structured probes of generalization, use of the trained verbal antecedents may give the desired information on generalization across a number of parameters. For probes of spontaneous production in natural environments, however, use of the same verbal antecedents used in training can easily result in misleading estimates of generalization.

In addition to using trained verbal antecedents to collect structured generalization data, language generalization research frequently does not report the verbal antecedents of language targets when natural-environment generalization is measured. When reading these reports, we assume that the target was uttered in appropriate contexts, i.e., after particular verbal or nonverbal antecedent events. What those events were may be described in general terms, but researchers rarely describe them specifically. When data must be gathered on a very specific target, waiting for that target to occur naturally may be quite time-consuming. However, accurate and rigorous measures of generalization of language target behaviors to natural environments requires that no planned verbal elicitation strategies be set up. Unobtrusive observations of clients interacting in their natural environments can reveal whether generalization programming *within* those environments may be necessary. If such observations reveal a failure to generalize, it may be necessary to teach persons in those environments to use particular verbal and visual antecedents to trigger or prompt the desired language behaviors.

THE PROBLEM OF SPONTANEOUS LANGUAGE

There are several ways of defining "spontaneous" language. Sometimes it is contrasted with "imitative" language and means simply language that is not the result of a request to repeat a model, such as, "Say 'This is a cat.' " Indeed, we can even observe "spontaneous" imitations, that is, repetitions of a model that were not elicited, or asked for. When spontaneous language refers only to nonimitated language, it includes answers to questions or directives that may have been used to teach the response in treatment programs.

A more stringent definition of "spontaneous" requires that the language be child-initiated rather than a response to a question or directive. Here, operationally defining spontaneous, child-initiated language becomes tricky, since conversational rules dictate that utterances be relevant to the topic, and thus utterances are usually responses to the previous speaker's language. One speaker may choose to initiate a new topic, but this usually occurs after a silence, a pause in the talk, or by use of a conversational device, such as "Oh, that reminds me. . . ." If our goal is to teach language so that the client produces it "spontaneously" in natural environments, we need a good definition of what we will consider "spontaneous" yet appropriately responsive to the topic of conversation. We also need more information on the kinds of verbal and visual antecedents that set the occasion or provide appropriate contexts for particular language behaviors, so that we can build these into our language teaching programs.

Since achieving appropriate spontaneous language is especially difficult in autistic individuals, it may be instructive to review some of the literature in autism that has addressed the issue of spontaneous language. In reporting generalization measures with autistic children, Lovaas and associates (1973) described a sampling condition in which an adult attended visually to the child, but did not comment or initiate any interaction with the child. Thus, any child language was spontaneous in the strictest sense, i.e., child-initiated.

In discussing strategies to teach spontaneous-functional speech to autistic children, Sosne, Handleman, and Harris (1979) advocate programs to reduce reliance on verbal prompts from others (e.g., "What's this?", "What do you see?", or "What do you want?") and to enhance the child's awareness of the physical environment as containing cues for speech. For teaching children to initiate conversation, the following six steps are suggested by Sosne and colleagues (1979): (1) create a need for speech by engineering the environment to facilitate speech; (2) establish the response, avoiding excessive verbal and nonverbal prompts; (3) program generalization by training across a variety of settings with different stimuli and trainers; (4) introduce and require advanced language by setting up conditions in which elaborated language is necessary to accomplish the desired goal; (5) establish communicative peer interactions with other children, using normal children and siblings, and (6) program in the home, with parents applying the general principles for facilitating spontaneous speech during normal household routines. These suggestions clearly are appropriate for teaching spontaneous language to nonautistic children as well.

It may also be useful to remember that we should expect a time gap between the production of language targets as *responses* and production of them as child-initiated or spontaneous language. For example, children acquiring Bliss symbols used the symbols initially in an exclusively respondent manner (Harris et al., 1979). Within two years, however, children were also using the symbols to initiate and interact spontaneously. A two-year gap may or may not be typical—expect the usual individual variation among language-handicapped clients.

Another way to avoid the problem of language targets that are produced only in response to verbal antecedents used in training is to fade the verbal cues and get the target to occur in response to the visual antecedent alone. However, this method can result in artificial-sounding language, a sign of stimulus-response conditioning rather than naturally produced speech about objects or events in the environment. Consider the anecdote reported by Rees (1978, p. 193) concerning the response of a mentally retarded girl to a cup: "It's a cup, it's pink, it's plastic, you drink out of it." Obviously, "spontaneous language" (in this case probably a response to a visual stimulus) is not necessarily appropriate to the context.

Examples of Verbal Antecedents

When the verbal antecedents used to teach language targets in some behavioral experimental literature are examined, two characteristics can be found that are now viewed as detrimental to generalization. Contrary to the principles of teaching more than one example and making the treatment environment similar to the natural environment, language targets are often taught by repeating the same verbal antecedent to elicit the response until criterion is met. While some may argue that this is necessary if the child is to learn the response at all, others would argue that if generalization rather than simply establishing the target is the goal, more varied antecedents should be used.

The other characteristic common to behavioral research on language teaching is selecting targets that are not particularly functional. These often require verbal antecedents that are not common in natural environments, another violation of generalization principles. For example, Handleman's (1979) research on children's learning of responses to questions and on generalization across settings used test questions such as, "What do you smell with?" and "Where do you take a bath?"

Perhaps these verbal antecedents would be appropriate for generalization to test situations in other school rooms, but they are hardly the kinds of questions that occur in most natural environments.

There are other behavioral studies of language teaching, however, that offer good examples of the application of principles that foster generalization, for example, the Campbell and Stremel-Campbell (1982) study describing a "loose" training program for teaching *is* and *are*. One of these generalization principles is to use multiple and diverse verbal antecedents to make the treatment conditions similar to those of natural environments. The specific words or phrases that precede target responses, or opportunities for target responses, in the natural environment vary widely. Questions or directives spoken by the classroom teacher often are not the same as those spoken by parents or siblings at home.

The language clinician faces a dilemma—whether to teach responses to a limited number of "canned" questions and directives, to visual antecedents only, or to a wide variety of verbal and visual antecedents, systematically varied in some pattern. The choice of which antecedents to use may vary with the individual client, the goal(s), and the stage of intervention. The cognitive capacities of the client may constrain the goals chosen as well as the variety of antecedent events to be used in training. During the establishment phase of language teaching, choosing only a few frequently occurring verbal antecedents may be the appropriate strategy. As learning progresses, more and varied combinations of verbal and visual antecedents should be used.

When the language target has been specified in speech act categories, such as requesting, commenting, or answering, the kinds of verbal antecedents that may accompany nonverbal contexts can be narrowed down to some that are probably used by talkers in the natural environment. Examples for facilitating requesting behaviors include indirect models, such as "If you want more colors, let me know" or "I'll get the scissors if you want them," and general statements, such as "This book looks like it might be fun to read" or "We could make a snowman" (Olswang, Kriegsmann, and Mastergeorge, 1982). In addition, these authors suggest presenting a visual antecedent, i.e., some kind of obstacle, such as a barrier or an absent object, along with a verbal directive. Examples include "Please pour the juice" (when the juice container can't be opened by the child), "Push the truck" (when the truck is broken), and "Finish the puzzle" (when a piece is missing). These suggestions constitute an effective pairing of both verbal and visual antecedents.

The combining of verbal and nonverbal antecedents is also illustrated by three suggestions offered by Hart (1981). In discussing the implications of recent research in developmental pragmatics for working with developmentally disabled children, Hart makes several points regarding the choice of antecedent events to use for promoting language generalization. The first relates to the importance of context, the second emphasizes generalized imitation, and the third proposes increasing the rate (frequency) of language use.

A frequent and pervasive cue that adults automatically present to normal speakers to trigger some kind of language response is often a delay—the adult maintains eye-contact and waits attentively for the person to speak. This signals conversational partners that it is their turn to talk. One of the first goals of language therapy, then, should be to train the child to recognize this cue and to respond, for example, with a verbal (or nonverbal, if necessary) request.

What do normal language users do when they wait, but no one responds to the cue of delay? A predictable prompt when the person seems to want something would be a question, for example: "What do you want?" or "Can I help you?" Hart makes the point here that two different responses should be taught—one for the delay cue (e.g., a statement or request) and one for the question (e.g., an elliptical answer)—because a full sentence is not expected in response to "What do you want?" Initially, of course, a single-word response would be appropriate for both cues.

Once the child has learned some appropriate responses to these two cues (delay and question) in therapy, the natural environment, or "everyday context" in Hart's terms, should be changed. This entails changing the behavior of both the child and the adults, who are probably responding to the child's inappropriate ways of communicating. Thus, the importance of context—that is, the everyday context of the natural environment—is emphasized from the outset of therapy.

The second of Hart's suggestions, teach or foster generalized imitation, is important if children are to learn new skills without direct teaching. What do adults do when confronted with a new situation in which they are unsure how to talk or act? They watch what others do in those situations and match their own behavior to what others are doing. They learn a contextual script by attending to who says what, how, when, and to whom. Thus, Hart recommends teaching children routines or interactional scripts for how to behave both nonverbally and verbally in given situations. The notion of generalized imitation parallels the notion of observational learning proposed by Bandura, the principle on which modeling studies of language intervention are based (see Chapter 3).

The third important suggestion made by Hart (1981) is to increase the rate of language use, because with increased rate comes increased elaboration. As Hart puts it, "...Given that language is appropriately matched to context, the more a person talks the more varied is the language used, not only because a person who talks a lot is likely to be commenting on a variety of objects, events, and relationships within the context, but because the context controlling language use changes in subtle ways with every utterance introduced into that context" (p. 309). This suggestion to increase rate is one of the principles of incidental teaching, discussed earlier in Chapter 3.

Initially, the clinician may have to prompt child language, either verbally or with a delay. To shape true initiation, the clinician may move away, or look away momentarily, so that the child's language functions to call attention to his or her message. Initially, too, the clinician must ensure that every child utterance functions appropriately, e.g., gets adult attention and is not ignored. Throughout the process, it is crucial that the immediate context of the interaction control the language that is used, for only in this way is an appropriate match maintained between context and language use.

Some generalization strategies similar to those suggested by Hart have been suggested by Culatta and Page (1982). A number of techniques designed to encourage spontaneous use of trained grammatical rules in natural settings are presented, and the emphasis is on communicative functions in natural contexts. Three types of generalization strategies are provided. The first is providing *reasons* to communicate—both to initiate communication and to use a specific grammatical language target. The second strategy is eliminating discriminative stimuli, i.e., those prompts and cues that occur frequently in structured therapy but rarely in natural environments. For example, disguising demands for specific grammatical targets and varying the communicative situations may decrease dependence on a discriminative stimulus as a reminder to produce the language target. The third strategy is using modeling and expansion within the clinician's language to increase exposure to and emphasize the grammatical feature targeted.

Culatta and Page (1982) provide some interesting examples of treatment sessions designed to foster production of grammatical targets within naturalistic conversational settings. For instance, to provide multiple opportunities for negative constructions, they suggest role-playing a scene where "mommy and daddy ... found a skunk in their garage ... (and) they've gotta find a way to get the skunk out" (p. 38). A reason to communicate, using negative constructions, has been provided in an indirect way that disguises requests for negatives and that allows the clinician to model negative sentences.

In their discussions of generalization strategies, neither Hart (1981) nor Culatta and Page (1982) addressed the role of consequences for correct and incorrect production of grammatical targets in their discussion of generalization strategies. Their focus was primarily on manipulation of antecedent events to increase the similarity between treatment and generalization conditions.

SAMPLE STUDIES

In view of the relative absence of studies that have directly investigated the effects of specific antecedent events on language target generalization, the following studies have been selected for readers to consider the role played by various antecedent events and the choice of language targets. Consider the studies described in the following sections. What are the verbal and visual antecedents for the language targets? What can clinicians learn about providing verbal and nonverbal antecedents that will promote generalization to natural environments? The following studies illustrate the use of verbal antecedents to trigger the occurrence of trained responses either to nontraining stimuli or within nontraining settings.

Object Label Training

One of the first language targets chosen for clients at a one-word stage is object labels. Initially, labels for desired objects may be taught not simply to name things, but to function as requests for those objects. The antecedent may be the sight of the object or the verbal prompt, "What do you want?" Later, the label may be produced in answer to a test question or even a sincere information question, such as "What's this?" or "What have you made?" In the following section, results of several descriptive and experimental studies are described, as they relate to teaching object labels so as to promote generalization of those labels.

The generalized effects of object label training with six severely retarded institutionalized children have been reported by Warren, Rogers-Warren, Baer, and Guess (1980) and by Warren and Rogers-Warren (1983a, 1983b). Object labels included names for food (milk, candy, apple), body parts (nose, tummy), eating utensils (cup, spoon), toys (ball), furniture (table), and clothes (shoe). Systematic language training programs (Guess, Sailor, and Baer, 1978; Stremel and Waryas, 1974) were administered for a total of 36 words, which varied in number for each child. The children also received six hours of daily classroom instruction in pre-academic, art, vocational, and self-help skills. An average of 15 labels was successfully trained to criterion in an average of 43 sessions. Structured probes within the classroom consisted of an adult asking, "What's this?" and presenting an item, twice. Verbal praise followed correct responses, whereas incorrect answers were ignored. Three of the children showed 100 per cent correct answers to probes, and the other three showed 69 to 95 per cent correct answers.

Once a word had been displayed in response to the structured probes, its occurrence in the natural environment was observed. Observations were made in two classrooms, dining hall, and living unit, with four to six language samples collected each week. Verbatim transcripts of the child's speech and speech directed to the child were made for the 15-minute periods. Both on-line transcription and tape recordings made via a transmitter in the child's apron were used for sample collections. Transcripts were computer-analyzed to chart the occurrence of trained and untrained words and to maintain a dictionary of each child's current vocabulary. Only nonimitated productions were considered for these generalization measures, but it was not clear whether labels occurred with or without the "What's this?" question, nor was it clear whether both requesting and labeling functions were included. Generalization ratios (number correct divided by total opportunities to occur) were computed for two conditions: each trained word occurring once and each trained word occurring twice. With the one-occurrence criterion, the six children averaged 79 per cent generalization of the trained labels; with the two-occurrence criterion, 66 per cent of the trained labels were considered to have generalized. For one child, only 18 per cent of the labels generalized to two occurrences. Thus, the more stringent criterion of two spontaneous productions in the natural environment resulted in apparently less generalization.

Of the 36 words trained, 16 were trained with three or more children, and 12 of these were successfully generalized by more than half the children. What kinds of words generalized best? Analyses of these words revealed labels that were or were not functional or useful for the children. We may infer that the words that showed the greatest generalization were the most functional for the retarded children in their institutional setting. Those words most likely to be generalized were names for foods, toys, eating utensils, and clothes. Furniture and body part names did not generalize well.

As Warren and colleagues discussed these results, the problems in data collection were elaborated. Since 15-minute samples taken four to six times per week can capture only a small fraction of the opportunities for appropriate use of object labels, the data collected may not be representative of the child's actual production of trained labels. If the verbal antecedent "What's this?" was used in the natural environment, one could question its sincerity. Would adult staff members in an institution ask a child for an object label unless they had been requested to do so as a probe for generalization across setting and person? The question "What's this?" is either an artificial question to test the listener's label knowledge or a sincere request for a label that is not known to the speaker—an unlikely question to be addressed to a retarded child, unless adults in the environment had been instructed to do so.

Alternatively, if occasions to produce object labels in natural environments, which included classrooms, dining hall, and living unit, were not prompted by questions, labels may have occurred as requests or comments when children saw a trained object. It would be interesting to know what verbal or visual antecedents triggered production of the trained object labels for the six children in the natural environments studied. Perhaps more study of the language addressed to institutionalized clients would help us decide what words to teach and which verbal antecedents to use in teaching word production in these settings.

A subsequent report on the same data (Warren and Rogers-Warren, 1983b) addressed the question of setting generalization more specifically, analyzing the labels produced in the three environments and the adult interactions occurring in each. The classroom was the setting in which most generalization occurred; e.g., 74 per cent more of the generalized words were used in the classroom than in either the dining hall or living unit.

While some of the labels occurred more frequently in one setting because of the nature of that setting (e.g., *apple, milk, spoon,* and *cookie* were repeatedly used in the dining hall), no correlational patterns were found between types of words that generalized and any setting. Rather, the verbal interactions in the classroom were fundamentally different from those observed in the other settings. Both the rate of adult verbalizations to subjects and the occasions when subjects were obligated to respond verbally to a question or command were highly correlated with the percent of generalization observed in each setting. Warren and Rogers-Warren suggest that the single greatest factor in achieving generalization of noun usage in each setting was the verbal behavior of the adults present. The interaction opportunities of the dining hall and living unit did not demand or support language usage by the retarded subjects. Thus, the trained labels generalized at relatively low rates in these environments.

The implications of these studies on generalization of noun labels are important for clinicians teaching initial vocabulary words to language-disordered individuals. The selection of functional words that will *need* to be used in natural environments is critical, as is the training of potential attentive listeners available in natural environments. Unless there are listeners whose attention can be gained and directed by the language-disordered individual's utterance of labels, trained labels are unlikely to generalize. Thus, both the content for language targets and the environmental support for those language targets must be considered when planning treatment programs with generalization in mind.

MULTIWORD COMBINATION TRAINING

When the language target consists of two or more word utterances, syntactic rules for word order must be taught. Training is done on one or a few combinations, and generalization to similar combinations is assessed. The goal is to teach the underlying rule (e.g., [noun + verb] or [agent + action]) rather than the surface form (e.g., "doggie eat"). The words in the child's vocabulary must include a sufficient number of nouns and verbs (or agents and actions) so that training can use some but not all of them, leaving some untrained vocabulary with which to test for generalization to untrained exemplars. Structured probes may be constructed to elicit various combinations, such as trained noun + untrained verb, untrained noun + trained verb, and untrained noun + untrained verb. Thus, generalization patterns on structured probes may be systematically measured. However, in spontaneous probes of conversational speech, a fourth combination can also be observed for two-word utterances, i.e., the trained noun + trained verb. In reporting generalization data, it would be important to include a breakdown of combination types, so that teaching strategies could be altered if certain patterns were not being generalized.

Some syntactic classes do not contain many possible exemplars (pronouns, for example), while other classes may contain a very large number (nouns, for example). Thus, some syntactic strings may be taught, which include *some* words that rarely change and one word that often changes. For instance, the request "I want *X*" includes two words that seldom vary (as long as intent remains the same) and one word that will vary depending on the item desired. A question arises here as to just how much change should be required in order to constitute evidence of generalization. A stringent criterion would require that multiple examples from each word class must be produced before the resulting behavior is called "generalization." Using the previous example, we'd want to hear "You like apple" and "They hate peas," as well as "I want cookie" before we would say a child has a syntactic rule for [pronoun + state-verb + noun]. In addition, we'd want to know whether such utterances were prompted with a *wh-* question such as "What do you want?" or were uttered without verbal prompting but in appropriate situations, before we would agree that the child is showing the desired generalized language behavior.

Generalization and Syntax Targets

An early report of generalization effects subsequent to syntax training showed disappointing results when more stringent criteria for generalization were applied (Warren et al., 1980). After training on 12 syntactic forms via the Guess, Sailor, and Baer (1978) program, four retarded subjects showed a mean of four forms generalized to the natural environment (33 per cent) over approximately seven months. After similar training on 23 forms, four language-delayed (nonretarded) preschool children showed a mean of five forms generalized (22 per cent). The investigators concluded at this point that changes in the forms chosen for training and the manner in which they were trained might have resulted in greater generalization.

However, a subsequent report on language generalization by six severely retarded institutionalized individuals who had received training via the Guess, Sailor, and Baer program for an average of 23 months (range of 16 to 31 months) provided more encouraging results (Warren and Rogers-Warren, 1983a). Data were analyzed separately for two-word, three-word, and four-word syntactic forms and for generalization to both classroom settings and dining room and living units. Of the 73 syntactic forms trained to criterion, 41 (56 per cent) generalized to the subjects' actual usage repertoires observed in natural environments, using the criterion of nonimitative production on at least two occasions. Data revealed that the shorter forms generalized best, i.e., 88 per cent of the two-word forms generalized, 66 per cent of the three-word forms generalized, and 32 per cent of the four-word forms generalized. The overall spontaneous MLU (mean length of utterance) of the group across the study was 1.8 morphemes. The overall MLU of the generalized forms was 2.8 morphemes, which was closer to the group's spontaneous MLU than the MLU of 3.5 for the nongeneralized forms. The greater generalization of shorter forms was demonstrated regardless of the function of the utterance (i.e., question, request, or answer). Results similar to these, which were obtained from severely mentally retarded subjects, were observed for mildly language-delayed preschool children (Warren, Rogers-Warren, and Buchanan, 1981). The MLU of successfully generalized forms was 2.8, whereas the subjects' overall MLU was 2.4 morphemes. Forms more than one morpheme greater than a child's average everyday speech did not generalize. Thus, it appears that an important factor to consider for fostering generalization would be to use what has been called a horizontal approach to language training, that is, teaching many different forms at the same MLU level rather than teaching longer and more complex forms. While subjects could learn these longer forms within the structured training sessions, the forms did not generalize well to natural environments. In general, training longer forms did not result in an overall increase in the group's MLU, since the longer forms did not generalize.

How long did it take for the trained forms to occur within the nonteaching environments observed? Again, the length of the target form seemed to be a factor. The two-word forms appeared in the generalization data approximately two weeks (8 observations) after criterion was achieved in training sessions. The four-word forms that generalized, on the other hand, did not appear until after 16 or more observations. Thus, not only did fewer four-word forms generalize, but the ones that did generalize were relatively slow to do so.

The generalization data collected within different settings for the Warren and Rogers-Warren (1983b) study showed relatively little setting effect on generalization. Although more forms generalized to the classroom setting (90 per cent of the generalized forms) than to the dining hall and living unit (78 per cent of the generalized forms), there was no systematic pattern among forms that failed to generalize to the three settings. Subjects talked more in the classroom than in the other two settings, and shorter utterances were used more than longer utterances in all three settings. Apparently, the forms were useful for the subjects in all three settings.

One other important result was found in this study by Warren and Rogers-Warren (1983b) that bears on generalization of language training. Correlational analyses revealed that subjects who talked more frequently in the nonteaching environments progressed faster through the training program and that subjects who talked more used longer and more diverse utterances. However, there was little relationship between frequency of talking and success at generalizing forms beyond the subject's current MLU range. Thus, while increasing the frequency of talking may be a primary goal for language-handicapped individuals, the clinician will still need to be cautious about teaching language targets that are well beyond the developmental level of the client.

Generalization and Semantic and Pragmatic Targets

The same data analyzed for evidence of generalization of syntactic forms in the initial report by Warren and co-workers (1980) were reanalyzed to examine generalization of the semantic relations expressed by those forms and for communicative function of the utterance. For two mildly delayed children who had been trained with multiple exemplars of each semantic relationship, strong generalization effects for five of the seven semantic relations were shown. However, the one severely retarded child displayed no syntactic or semantic generalization. Concurrent with training on nine different exemplars of the control function, a strong acceleration in the use of control statements was demonstrated for one child. This child used *untrained* syntactic forms to control the environment. Again, the retarded child did not show any increase in the control function as a result of training.

The data reported by Warren and colleagues (1980) suggest that generalization of correct syntax is a more difficult skill than is generalization of object labels or communicative functions such as requesting. The greater generalization across semantic relations suggests that early language-rule learning occurs across semantic, not syntactic, categories—a phenomenon found in normally developing children acquiring their first language. The successful generalization of the control function of language, expressed with various exemplars, also parallels the development of communicative functions in normal children, e.g., the protoimperatives described by Bates, Camaioni, and Volterra (1975). It may be that selection of early language goals based on the results of developmental research on the normal population would result in more successful training of language within disordered populations. Systematic research is needed to determine the conditions of generalization failure and generalization success. Only such controlled research can reveal the efficiency of various language-training sequences (Brinker and Bricker, 1979).

VERBAL ANTECEDENTS IN CONVERSATIONS

For adult mentally retarded individuals, a frequent target of language therapy may be conversational skills, rather than specific vocabulary or grammar targets. One of the major cues for appropriate conversation is the verbal antecedent. Thus, in teaching conversational skills it is important to pay attention to the verbal antecedents typical in conversational interaction and to teach appropriate responses to them. Several examples of social skills training programs have emphasized the conversational aspects of social skills, and some of them are described in subsequent chapters. The following studies offer some considerations for choosing antecedent events for conversational responses.

A descriptive study of the verbal interactions between staff and residents in an institutional setting revealed some interesting data relevant for teaching conversational skills (Prior, Minnes, Coyne, Golding, Hendy, and McGillivary, 1979). The verbal interactions occurring between 29 mentally retarded residents, ranging in age from 8 to 32 years, and 11 staff persons were categorized and statistically analyzed. Categories for staff verbal initiations were Comment, Instruction, Question, and Conversation (defined as utterances directly solicitous of an extended informative response or representing a normal attempt at initiating a conversation). Only two categories, Incomprehensible and Verbal, were used for resident verbal initiations. Categories for staff and resident responses were Ignore, Acquiescent Nonverbal, Yes-No, Question, Comment, and Conversation. Interaction in both structured (dining room and occupational therapy room) and unstructured (day recreation room, outside) settings was observed. Results indicated that the most frequent staff initiation was Instruction (e.g., "Go and sit down"), and the least frequent was Conversation (e.g., "What did you do today?"). Unfortunately, the least frequent staff initiation, Conversation, was the most favorable form of communication for promoting verbal responses from residents. When residents verbally initiated, staff ignored those initiations approximately one third of the time. Such responses can be considered nonreinforcing and probably result in a decreased frequency of verbal initiations. Structured settings were more likely to encourage language use than were unstructured settings.

Clinicians who work at or consult for institutions for the mentally retarded may find these data useful for providing in-service information to personnel or for involving staff in programs designed to increase generalization of conversational skills. Two groups of language targets may need to be considered. Appropriate language targets or skills must be selected for particular clients who live within a residential setting or work in sheltered workshop settings. In addition, particular language targets may be selected for the potential listeners and conversational partners who will interact with clients in these special settings. For generalization to be achieved, it may be necessary to address the language behaviors of both clients and personnel within residential and work environments.

The problem of getting trained language behavior to occur within conversational discourse, though not within a nontreatment setting, was investigated by Culatta and Horn (1982). Subjects were four language-disordered children who could produce their grammatical targets with 100 per cent accuracy in response to clinically structured tasks designed to evoke them. Analysis of their spontaneous language revealed correct target production in only 50 to 70 per cent of the obligatory contexts that occurred. The experimental design was a multiple baseline across two targets for each child. Targets included the verbs *is, am, will*, and *went*, the pronoun *he*, and the negative *not*. Teaching procedures included role-playing of real-world events with dolls and objects and verbal and nonverbal strategies to evoke the grammatical targets many times within each session.

The program began with a high density of clinician-modeled utterances and evoking situations (75 per cent), and progressed toward a lower density (less than 25 per cent) of these therapy procedures. All subjects successfully reached 90 to 100 per cent criterion production by the completion of 19 to 27 twice-weekly sessions of 45 minutes. Probes at least seven sessions after training stopped on the first target showed that these targets were maintained at a 90 per cent accuracy rate. However, since spontaneous discourse data were always collected within the treatment sessions, perhaps the term *maintenance* is misleading. It was not clear whether children were also correctly producing their grammatical targets in spontaneous discourse outside the clinical setting when talking to a variety of listeners.

One other study of pragmatic behaviors, which included a generalization measure, also addresses the issue of verbal antecedents used for treatment and generalization measures. This research also describes an interesting procedure for treating conversational language behaviors (Gajar, Schloss, Schloss, and Thompson, 1984). Two youths who had suffered head trauma, whose conversational skills were inappropriate, were treated by alternate phases of feedback and self-monitoring treatments. The clients were part of a four-person group, which participated in sessions with a facilitator who followed a standard protocol. In the clinic room, sessions began with the facilitator reading a "Dear Abby" column twice, then asking, "Are there any questions?" Concurrent with the treatment sessions, two other facilitators conducted a less structured group session in a client lounge, with conversation initiated by asking, "What shall we talk about today?" Data from this session constituted the generalization measure. Thus, the verbal antecedents used to assess generalization across persons and settings differed. For both treatment and generalization sessions, facilitators waited 3 seconds before beginning a prompting hierarchy of questions. Positive responses included relevant statements, agreement or disagreement with a previous statement, or relevant questions. Negative responses included silence after a question or statement, three or fewer words, off-topic or mumbled responses, jokes, or interruptions.

During the feedback phase, observers behind a one-way mirror operated a toggle switch that caused a green light (for positive conversational behaviors) or a red light (negative conversational behaviors) to be displayed on a unit visible to the group members. During the self-monitoring phase, the toggle switches were controlled by the group members. For comparison purposes, data were collected from two groups of normal college students meeting for the first time. The format for one group paralleled that of the treatment session, and the format for the other group paralleled that of the generalization session.

Results of this study indicated that both feedback and self-monitoring had positive effects on the conversational behaviors of the two clients (Gajar et al., 1984). Rates of positive conversational behaviors were higher in all treatment phases in comparison to baseline phases. Both intervention approaches brought rates into the ranges observed in normal students. For one client, the self-monitoring treatment was more effective, but for the other client, the feedback treatment was more effective. Generalization data provided evidence that treatment gains had a positive effect in the less structured group situation, indicating some generalization across setting and persons.

The study by Gajar and co-workers offers a protocol for measuring and scoring conversational behaviors and is also quite encouraging in terms of the generalization observed. This study also illustrates an effective way to determine what might be considered an appropriate level of pragmatic behaviors. The data provided by the assessment of normal students' rates of positive and negative conversational behaviors were used to judge treatment and generalization effectiveness. It would be interesting to apply the feedback and self-monitoring approaches with other clients who exhibit conversational skill deficiencies.

NONVERBAL ANTECEDENTS

In considering what kinds of visual antecedents to use in both establishing a language target and facilitating generalization of it, a number of attributes might be considered. Several studies have compared objects with pictures as visual stimuli for teaching words. Other aspects of the nonverbal context that may influence language target production and generalization include the newness or novelty of the examples used, the presence of obstacles or barriers to desired objects, and other features of the nonlinguistic contexts that elicit language in natural environments.

The choice of picture or object stimuli may be influenced by a number of factors, such as the age or cognitive level of the client, and the ultimate goal of therapy. It has often been suggested that younger children, or clients at early cognitive levels, attend better to objects and thus may learn better given object stimuli. Picture stimuli, or photographs, can more easily represent a wide variety of referents, however, and if the goal is vocabulary teaching, picture stimuli may be a good choice. If pictures are to be used, however, we must ensure that the label is also transferred to the real object represented in the picture.

A study described in more detail in Chapter 5 compared three stimulus modalities (picture-cards, photographs, and real objects) on their effectiveness at achieving generalization of naming responses to real objects in the natural environment (Welch and Pear, 1980). Three of the four retarded children displayed considerably more generalization when they were trained with real objects, whereas the fourth child show substantial generalization regardless of the training stimulus mode. Subsequent research with one child showed that simultaneous use of picture-cards and real objects facilitated transfer from pictures to real objects for later trained names. The results of this study suggest that real objects should be used initially in teaching names (labels) for objects and that pairing pictures with objects for a time may facilitate eventual transfer from picture to object modalities.

Less clear-cut results were observed for four autistic children in a picture-versus-object comparison study by Handleman, Powers, and Harris (1984). Rather than assessing generalization to real objects in the natural environment, generalization to the alternate form of stimulus presentation was assessed by structured probes, following achievement of criterion on the trained form. Results indicated no consistent functional relationship between the two types of stimulus presentation, and there were varying degrees of generalization between the two forms. None of the subjects demonstrated complete (100 per cent) generalization from one form to the other, but all four boys generalized some names to the alternate form. In discussing their results, Handleman and co-workers emphasized the individual nature of generalization problems demonstrated by severely developmentally delayed children and also cautioned against assuming that names learned for pictures will automatically generalize to the objects those pictures represent.

The novelty of the stimulus items is another aspect of visual and other nonlinguistic stimuli that must be considered in teaching language to facilitate generalization. This variable may be particularly important in the establishment phase of language learning, but it also has implications for eliciting language targets in natural environments when assessing generalization. In a study of mentally retarded children at the one-word production stage, Leonard, Cole, and Steckol (1979) found that children were significantly more likely to imitate words when those words referred to unfamiliar and informative items, rather than to unchanging, noninformative items. These results suggest that in choosing both verbal and visual antecedents to use in teaching language targets, clinicians should consider the novelty of the example (e.g., they should frequently introduce new toys, objects, and events) and the informativeness of those antecedents (e.g., they should sequence the presentation of examples so that the target is a change from a series of previous examples). These suggestions support the Stokes and Baer advice to "teach multiple exemplars."

The novelty of certain visual stimuli is used to teach question-asking behavior via the Guess, Sailor, and Baer program (1978). When known items are presented, the client is to label them, but when unknown items are presented, the client is to ask, "What's that?" A study of the generalization and maintenance of such question-asking behavior in severely retarded institutionalized individuals was reported by Warren, Baxter, Anderson, Marshall, and Baer (1981) and provides another example of nonverbal antecedent events for a specific language target. The eight subjects studied had achieved criterion on the question target an average of 30 months prior to the study.

A generalization probe consisting of presentation of a brown bag or box was used to assess generalization of "What's that?" The container was shaken after 15 seconds, if no response occurred, and three different containers were used for the probes. Two of the eight subjects responded with "What's that?" or "What's in there?," showing generalization of the target across time. These two subjects showed significantly higher test scores on the Houston Test for Language Development (Crabtree, 1963) than did the remaining subjects. The remaining six subjects were exposed to a peer model who was reinforced for asking "What's that?" while the subject observed. For two of the six subjects, exposure to three to six peer models was successful in reestablishing the response to the "brown bag." However, the four remaining subjects required some retraining (one to three sessions) under conditions of the original training, i.e., 30-trial sessions with known and novel objects, before they were able to ask the question successfully during the brown bag generalization probe.

The use of the containers to set up a high-curiosity situation was a more naturalistic and probably more difficult test of generalization than the structured probes used as part of the original training. Thus, it is not surprising that generalization across time was not demonstrated by all eight subjects. Indeed, it is encouraging that little extra training was needed to reestablish the question response. The authors suggest that time itself is not a major factor in extinction of a trained language behavior, but that sufficiency of training and the function of the response in the natural environment are the prime determinants of generalization (Warren et al., 1981).

EFFECTIVE COMBINING OF VERBAL AND NONVERBAL ANTECEDENTS

One of the general principles of promoting generalization is to make the conditions of treatment and the natural environment similar. When conditions are similar, the client is less likely to discriminate between the treatment and natural environments and produce the target behavior only under treatment conditions. Applying this principle to the selection of verbal and visual antecedents to use in teaching language, we may consider the conditions under which the language targets are used in nontreatment situations. The characteristic of diversity of verbal antecedents was presented earlier. The variety of visual or nonverbal antecedents for language target production should also be stressed. However, taken together, the verbal and nonverbal events that set the occasion for a particular language response may be highly predictable. If clinicians can teach the salient features of both verbal and nonverbal antecedents, their clients can learn to produce language targets that are appropriate to those situational contexts. For some clients, depending on both cognitive and language developmental levels and characteristics of their natural environments, it may be advisable to teach routines, or scripts to follow, tailored to the specific situations frequently encountered in their sheltered environments, rather than to try to teach global language behaviors that may be suitable for other clients. Much of the current descriptive research on developmental pragmatics may provide ideas for setting up verbal and nonverbal contexts that might be expected to elicit particular language targets.

ANTECEDENT EVENTS IN INCIDENTAL TEACHING

Regardless of the strategy chosen, effective combining of both verbal and nonverbal events that precede language use in natural environments is necessary. One example of such effective pairing is illustrated by the incidental teaching approach of Hart and Risley (1982).

The procedure for language teaching called incidental teaching is the result of years of extensive research by Hart and Risley (1968, 1974, 1975) and Hart and Rogers-Warren (1978). Although the basic elements of incidental teaching have been used by effective teachers and parents for many years, the development of a consistent and systematic structure for teaching elaborate language that can be applied with empirically tested results has become available only recently. A brief manual, *How to Use Incidental Teaching for Elaborating Language* (Hart and Risley, 1982), outlines a series of nine steps in the procedure. Much of the initial research on incidental teaching techniques was carried out on disadvantaged preschool children, but the procedure has also been adapted for more severely language-delayed or disordered populations (Hart and Rogers-Warren, 1978), including autistic adolescents (McGee, Krantz, Mason, and McClannahan, 1983).

Early research in operant language training technology showed that such procedures were effective in training various aspects of language and speech in both institutional and preschool settings. However, generalization problems were noted; language trained under close stimulus control failed to generalize to any marked extent into spontaneous language use in uncontrolled situations (Hart and Risley, 1980). This realization prompted Hart and Risley to create conditions for the generalization of language behaviors taught in controlled training sessions to children's natural environments, one of which is the preschool classroom. The preschool environment was rearranged so that the trained language was not only functional but necessary for gaining access to reinforcers such as adult attention, materials, and activities. Results of an early study (Hart and Risley, 1968) indicated not only that generalization of a specific language behavior (use of adjectives) could be achieved by incidental teaching procedures, but that direct language training might be conducted effectively in the preschool classroom. Subsequent research confirmed that brief, one-to-one interactions between teacher and child, in an environment rich in attractive and accessible potential reinforcers, could result in successful "in vivo" teaching of generalized language behaviors.

Basic to the incidental teaching procedure is the child's initiation of communication. To increase the chances that such initiation will occur, the setting is arranged to include two crucial elements: something to talk about or request (attractive and appropriate materials and activities) and an adult whose attention and approval is important to the child and who will provide help with or permission for gaining access to the materials or activities. Once the interaction is initiated by the child, the teacher (parent, therapist) conducts incidental teaching by focusing close attention on the child and asking for elaborated language related to the topic the child has specified. If the child does not respond or responds incorrectly, a prompt appropriate for the child's language level is given. If this does not result in the desired language, a model is then provided, with a request for the child to repeat it. Finally, the teacher confirms the response, models the elaborated language, and gives the child what was asked for.

Users of incidental teaching are cautioned that the conditions appropriate for incidental teaching are not always in effect. Teaching adults must be sensitive to both the child's and their own readiness for conducting incidental teaching. The procedure is most enjoyable and effective when it is casually and briefly applied frequently through the day. Not only must decisions be made about when to use incidental teaching, but decisions concerning the child's topic, the best prompt to use, and the degree of elaboration of a language target to ask for must also be made. These decisions require some familiarity with the child's ability, and consultations with the speech-language clinician should provide classroom teachers and parents with necessary information concerning the best prompts and the kinds of language elaboration to expect.

One of the first results noted after incidental teaching procedures are applied with language-disordered children is a simple increase in frequency of talking (Hart and Risley, 1980; Rogers-Warren and Warren, 1980). Once the verbal output of a child increases, the opportunities to shape that output, to model elaborated sentences, and to apply specific consequences also increase. Thus, a treatment program that results in increased frequencies of talking provides increased opportunities for language teaching.

CONCLUSIONS

In summarizing this chapter on the characteristics of verbal and visual antecedents that may be conducive to generalization across various parameters, a number of specific suggestions are offered. Table 4–1 presents a brief list of suggestions, with examples for applying each, that have been derived from the research summarized in this chapter.

Table 4–1. Suggestions for Selecting Verbal and Visual Antecedents to Promote Generalization

1. Use a variety of verbal antecedents during the establishment phase.

   Example 1: As prompts to elicit verbal labels as single words or in sentences, use: "What's this?," "Gee, I don't know what this is," "I wonder what this is called . . .," or even "Bet you don't know what the name of this is . . ."

   Example 2: As prompts for sentences with adjectives, use: "Tell me about . . ." or "This little girl has never seen a _______ before. Would you describe one for her?"

Table 4–1 (*continued*).

Example 3: As prompts for explanations, use: "This little boy doesn't know how to _______. Could you tell him how to _______?"

2. Use a pause, and delay asking a question or commenting, in order to give the client a chance to initiate language. The pause may result in either a question or a comment from the client.

   Example 1: Cover up part of a picture and wait, to elicit some type of question.

   Example 2: Present a box or bag and wait, or take an unfamiliar or unusual object out of a bag and wait, to elicit a comment or question.

3. Follow the delay with a typical question that might be asked in natural environments, e.g., "Do you want something?" or "May I help you?"

4. Intersperse the presentation of new information (e.g., novel toys, objects, or pictures) with repeated presentations of old information.

   Example: Use four known objects, actions, attributes, or locations as teaching stimuli and randomly add a fifth unknown stimulus.

5. Teach responses to verbal antecedents paired with appropriate visual stimuli, then fade out the verbal prompt.

   Example: During role playing, provide pictured grocery items and prompt *where*-questions by stating, for example, "You need to find out where the orange juice is in this grocery store." Then fade the verbal prompt.

6. Use both pictures and objects as visual stimuli. Make sure that the language targets generalize to both modalities.

7. After language targets are learned as *responses* to a variety of antecedents, promote *spontaneous,* client-initiated production of appropriate language targets.

   Example 1: Move away and ignore the client so that language must be used to get your attention.

   Example 2: Set up situations designed to elicit comments, requests, questions, or other language targets, and wait while maintaining eye contact with the client.

Chapter 5
Stimulus Generalization Across Settings

One aspect of the stimulus complex in language therapy is the setting—a special therapy room, a special space within a classroom, perhaps a particular table and chairs. If the language target behavior is learned only in the treatment setting and fails to occur in nontreatment settings, then treatment cannot be considered very effective. Most language behaviors should occur in such generalization settings as the child's home, the adult client's living environment, various classroom settings, various work settings, and play environments.

Much language intervention research has included setting generalization as the major goal, or at least as one of several goals. For this chapter, studies of setting generalization have been grouped into etiological categories, including the mentally retarded, the autistic, and the language disordered (including language-delayed) populations. Readers may elect to skip certain sections, thinking that the clinical populations encountered in their work would not include some of these groups. However, strategies applied to one type of client may often yield useful ideas for work with other types of clients. While the settings to which generalization of language behaviors is desired may differ for various clients, the procedures for measuring setting generalization and the methods used to achieve it may be quite similar across the various client groups.

The generalization settings studied include classrooms, homes, various rooms within a group home, outdoors, and others. Consider the numerous nontreatment settings to which a client's language behavior can generalize.

STUDIES WITH THE MENTALLY RETARDED POPULATION

In this section six studies that included measures of setting generalization are summarized. Subjects ranged from profoundly mentally retarded institutionalized adults to moderately retarded children. Output modes included speech, sign, and Bliss symbols. Table 5–1 indicates the language behaviors, settings, and results for these studies.

Generalization of manual sign production across two settings was investigated by Duker and Morsink (1984), using four profoundly retarded individuals. Two institutionalized women in their 20's, with mental and social ages in the range of two to four years, were taught iconic signs. Signs were selected after observation of subjects' interest in various objects or activities. Signs were used as requests and included such objects and activities as playing with a pegboard, stringing beads, listening to or making music, cleaning, and opening/closing doors. Signs were trained in a multiple-baseline design, across signs.

A transfer of stimulus control procedure was used, whereby imitation of the modeled sign was replaced by sign production in response to verbal instruction with no manual model. Teaching steps included physical guidance for sign production, which was subsequently faded, followed by imitation of a sign model, which was also subsequently faded. Training continued until each subject had mastered four signs—approximately 60 sessions of 20 minutes each, conducted five days per week. Generalization probes were collected from the beginning of training. Twice-weekly classroom probes were conducted by the teacher, who presented verbal instructions only. Ward probes were conducted by an available ward staff member once each week. Thus, this study investigated generalization across both settings and persons.

Results indicated that acquisition of the first sign required the longest time (16 and 19 sessions); subsequent signs were acquired more rapidly. Generalization of responding to verbal instructions within classroom and ward settings also occurred sooner with each additional sign. However, some signs were more likely than others to generalize across settings. A follow-up probe, conducted in all three settings (therapy-room, classroom, and ward) three months after the study revealed that one subject had maintained two of the four signs, and the other had maintained all four signs (Duker and Morsink, 1984).

Two additional retarded subjects, similar to those described above but younger, were trained such that visual stimuli (presentation of an object) rather than verbal stimuli controlled sign production. One of these subjects showed both retarded and autistic behaviors; both had experienced failure in previous attempts to have spoken words control motor behavior. Training procedures for these subjects did not include manual sign production in response to verbal instructions. Results showed a high degree of between-subject variation, with the child who was retarded-only achieving criterion levels very quickly and the other child requiring many more trials (e.g., 23 for the first sign). Generaliza-

Table 5–1. Studies of Setting Generalization with the Mentally Retarded (MR) Population

Authors	Subjects	Output Mode	Language Target	Settings	Results
Duker and Morsink (1984)	4 profoundly MR institutionalized adults	Signs	Requests for objects and activities, e.g., pegs for pegboard, listening to music	Training in TR*; probes to classroom and ward	Generalization across settings; some signs more likely to generalize than others
Welch and Pear (1980)	4 institutionalized MR children	Speech, Bliss symbols	Object labels for real objects, pictures, and photographs (e.g., kitchen utensils and toys)	Training in TR; probes in living area	More setting generalization for real objects than for pictures and photographs
Garcia, Bullet, and Rust (1977)	2 MR adolescents	Speech	Complex sentences, e.g., "If the dishes get dirty, then I will gather them and clean them all up."	Training in TR; probes to classroom and home	Failure to achieve generalization until training was introduced in nontherapy settings
Hegde and McConn (1981)	1 MR adult	Speech	Plural sentences with *are* in conversational speech	Training in TR; probes in occupational setting	Generalization at 69–80% until additional programming was applied in occupational setting
Foxx, McMorrow, and Mennemeier (1984)	6 institutionalized MR adults	Speech	Six social skills: compliments, social interaction, politeness, criticism, social confrontation, and questions/answers	Training in TR; probes in simulated and real workshops	Fair amount of generalization to simulated workshop; considerable variability in workshop setting; failure to generalize concluded
Campbell and Stremel-Campbell (1982)	2 moderately MR children	Speech	*Is* and *are* in 3 types of sentences: *wh-* questions, yes-no questions, and statements	Training in classroom during academic tasks; probes to free-play setting	Successful generalization across settings

*TR = Treatment room

tion to other settings and maintenance at three months were far better for the retarded-only child also (Duker and Morsink, 1984).

In discussing their study, Duker and Morsink stressed the high degree of between-subject variability, a general feature of performance within the mentally retarded population. However, they also suggested that the functional significance a sign has for the individual subject will probably affect both acquisition and generalization rates.

The Duker and Morsink study illustrates effective use of the advice of Stokes and Baer to "program common stimuli." When the activities and objects each subject was interested in were observed, target signs with a good probability of being learned were chosen. Thus, without including other persons in the training phase, some setting and person generalization was achieved, as well as some maintenance of sign production on a three-month follow-up measure.

Another study of setting generalization, this one using institutionalized retarded children, was conducted by Welch and Pear (1980), who compared picture cards, photographs, and real objects as modes of training stimuli for object-naming. The dependent variable for this within-subjects design was naming behavior in the natural environment, that is, the child's living area. The four subjects, all functioning at a two- to three-year level, received training within the training room on five different names with each of the three stimulus modes. Two used speech, one used Blissymbol pointing, and one used sign language to produce the object names. A pool of 58 stimuli represented common household items from categories such as kitchen utensils, bathroom items, clothing and accessories, toys, and tools. Edible reinforcers were used for all three stimulus modes. Names trained by use of real objects could show only setting generalization; names trained by pictures or photographs could show both stimulus mode and setting generalization.

Results showed that three of the four children displayed considerably more generalization to real objects in the natural environment when real objects were used in training. The fourth child showed substantial setting generalization regardless of the mode of training stimulus used. Supplementary procedures used with one child showed that training in several environments facilitated setting generalization to real objects, but only when real objects were used as training stimuli. Supplementary procedures also showed that transfer from picture-card to real-object stimuli was facilitated by pairing picture cards with the real objects portrayed by them.

This study by Welch and Pear (1980) demonstrates several of the Stokes and Baer suggestions for facilitating generalization. By selecting the names of common household items as the targets to be learned, the experimenters programmed common stimuli. By training in several different settings, they trained sufficient exemplars. However, reinforcement for correct responding (foods) was not a natural consequence of producing object names. In addition, the mere presentation or viewing of an object is a rather artificial stimulus for evoking a naming response.

This study has important implications for clinicians who train language responses, whether for articulation, grammar, or syntax remediation, by using picture-cards or photographs. When pictures or photographs are used, the clinician should be extremely careful and prompt in assessing generalization to real objects. If responses are stimulus-bound—that is, produced only when the picture or photograph is present but not when actual objects are present—a change in teaching tactics is necessary.

Setting generalization of a more complex language target was experimentally investigated by Garcia, Bullet, and Rust (1977). Two mentally retarded 16-year-olds were trained to respond with complex sentences (e.g., "If the dishes get dirty, then I will gather them and clean them all up") to action pictures and the verbal antecedent, "Tell me about this picture." By use of a multiple-baseline design, generalization of each sentence was monitored in a classroom by a male instructor and in the home by a parent. As failure was noted on generalization probes outside therapy, the instructor and parent were brought into the therapy room. When generalization did not result from this training with multiple persons, training (consequating responses) began in the classroom and home on only the first five words of the target sentence. This, too, failed to achieve generalization, and five more samples of the entire response were added to trials in the nontherapy settings, with training on one of the five. Results indicated that little generalization occurred, even though 100 per cent correct responding was observed in the therapy room. Not until training was introduced in the nontherapy settings, for the entire response, did generalization occur.

This study indicates that generalization across persons can be achieved, while setting generalization fails. It was evident that the *person* was not the controlling stimulus for either subject. In addition, training on only part of the language target in additional settings was not sufficient to achieve setting generalization. It appears that actual training within the settings where generalization is desired may be needed, at least for some subjects and some language targets.

Like most other generative responding studies, the study by Garcia and co-workers (1977) did not report whether the complex sentences generalized to spontaneous production in natural environments. The target structure, *if-then* complex sentences, may not be particularly useful or necessary for subjects to use in spontaneous conversational speech; thus, choice of language target may be questioned. The study was a good example, however, of well-controlled and systematic probes of generalization to nontherapy settings.

The need for systematic probes of generalization is illustrated in many studies. Only if we find out that generalization is not occurring at a desired rate, or across necessary parameters, can we add a specific strategy to the program designed to achieve a particular kind of generalization. For some clients and for some language behaviors, generalization programming may not be needed. However, many language behaviors trained in the mentally retarded population will probably require special programming to achieve generalization across settings.

An example of the addition of a generalization phase to the treatment program for a grammar target is found in Hegde and McConn's (1981) study of a retarded adult. After criterion had been reached for *are* production in sentences in treatment, generalization measures were collected in an occupational setting. Even though 94 to 98 per cent correct responding had been achieved in the treatment setting, conversational probes of *are* in the occupational setting showed 69 to 80 per cent correct production, an unacceptable rate for a grammatical target that should occur in 100 per cent of the obligatory contexts that occur during conversation. Application of a modest amount of reinforcing and punishing ("no") consequences to the subject's conversational speech within the occupational setting resulted in spontaneous use of the target in that setting.

Such additional programming after failure to generalize to a nontreatment setting has been discovered involved taking the treatment program out into one of the client's natural environments. Perhaps the same outcome (generalization to spontaneous production in an occupational setting) could have been achieved by incorporating appropriate generalization strategies (e.g., training in multiple settings) into the initial treatment program. Further research will be needed to find ways to predict which clients will require what kinds of generalization programming.

The training and generalization of verbal skills relevant to vocational settings was also investigated by Foxx, McMorrow, and Mennemeier (1984) within an institution for mentally retarded adults. Because of the difficulty in monitoring trained skills within natural settings, past social-skills research has used simulated situations to assess generalization, and such research has generally failed to demonstrate generalization. When simulated situations that approximate the natural setting have been used to assess generalization, events that artificially prime the trained behavior may be used, and natural stimulus events that trigger inappropriate verbal behavior may be excluded. Thus, the generalization observed may not be a true indication of the generalization that will occur within the natural environment. To address these issues, Foxx and colleagues used both a simulation and unobtrusive measures within the institution's workshop to assess generalization of trained verbal skills.

Two groups of three residents were trained in a multiple-baseline design across groups. The mildly or moderately retarded subjects, ranging in age from 19 to 41, were matched within each group. All could speak in complete sentences and had independent self-help skills. Target behaviors were six social skill areas: compliments, social interaction, politeness, criticism, social confrontation, and questions-answers. The commercially available board game *Sorry!* and an adapted set of 48 cards were used to teach the verbal skills. Both actor situations, which required players to initiate interactions, and reactor situations, which required players to respond to another's initiation, were included in the training. Scoring of responses was determined both by criteria developed earlier (Foxx, McMorrow, and Schloss, 1983) and by additional data obtained from mental health personnel. Data on nontarget behaviors, such as verbalizations as residents worked on a structured task, and productivity were collected daily by videotape recordings in the workshop. In addition to this naturalistic measure of generalization, pre- and post-simulations were conducted in a separate basement area set up to simulate the workshop, with a work area and a break area.

During training, individualized performance criteria were established, based on each subject's mean baseline performance. Criteria advanced from 30 per cent to 60 per cent, then to 90 per cent above the baseline mean. Following each game, subjects received a preselected reward if criterion was achieved. An undergraduate psychology student served as facilitator for 12 games for each group, providing specific positive and negative feedback for responses. Then the workshop supervisor conducted a four-game training series to assess whether the players' performance levels would be maintained and whether this technique would enhance generalization of appropriate verbal social behaviors to the workshop setting.

Results indicated that one group improved from a baseline average of 43 per cent correct responding to 77 per cent correct responding, while the other group improved from a baseline average of 39 per cent correct responding to 72 per cent correct responding. Both groups were responding near 90 per cent correct by the end of the 12 games. Individual analysis revealed that players' performance generally continued to improve as they were reexposed to each of the four card sequences. During the four games conducted by the workshop supervisor, performance for the first group averaged 88 per cent correct and for the second group, 76 per cent correct. Thus, generalization of trained verbal skills generalized to a second person.

The pre- and post-simulation assessments showed a fair amount of generalization to a simulated workshop condition. The first group's performance increased from 33 per cent to 63 per cent correct, and the second group's performance increased from 31 per cent to 62 per cent correct. The daily generalization measures collected in the workshop, however, were not so encouraging. There was considerable variability in both group and individual data. Although mean appropriate interactions increased from baseline to training periods, two subjects showed a downward trend in appropriate interactions. For the first group, the mean of appropriate interactions was actually lower during the supervisor training condition than during the earlier condition. For the second group, this mean was slightly increased. In addition to measures of appropriate interactions, mean number of words per response was also measured during baseline, 12-game, and 4-game periods. For the first group, mean words per response increased from 4.3 to 7.8 to 8.6 words across the three periods. For the second group, mean words per response increased from 4.8 to 5.3 to 6.2 words across the three periods. Thus, in addition to showing some generalization of appropriate verbal behaviors across settings and persons, a gross measure of language also showed improvement with training.

After the board game training was completed, videotape recording in the workshop continued once each week for a month. While there was again considerable variability in individual measures, both groups' follow-up performances averaged the same as or higher than appropriate interactions during the supervisor-conducted training games. Individual data showed that four of the six subjects' appropriate interactions were highest during follow-up.

Foxx, McMorrow, and Mennemeier (1984) concluded that although their results demonstrated support for the notion that training resulted in generalization to a simulated setting, generalization results in the actual workshop setting were equivocal. The variability of individual data both during baseline and during training, plus the downward trend in the training data of two subjects, indicated that the effects of the training program did not generalize. No experimental evidence demonstrated a functional relationship between any improved social responding and participation in the training program. In discussing these results, Foxx and colleagues suggested that the workshop setting contained stimulus variables, especially peers, that triggered inappropriate social behavior. Since both positive and negative social interactions are largely determined by the behavior of others, it is unlikely that improved verbal skills will generalize suddenly. As the investigators state, "...Residents with a long history of inappropriate interactions probably cannot be expected to begin interacting appropriately when they are placed together in a group assessment" (Foxx et al., 1984, p. 351). The need for inclusion of peers, as well as for conducting long-term generalization assessments in natural environments, was stressed for future research.

In view of suggestions for facilitating generalization, it would be fruitful to try application of the consequences—that is, the specific positive and negative feedback used during the games—to the verbal social interactions within the workshop setting in this study. Even though the supervisor apparently did apply these consequences during the four-game training series, there is no indication that the supervisor generalized these consequences to the actual workshop setting. Of course, if this treatment program had been used in the workshop setting, results could no longer be considered "automatic" generalization, but "programmed" generalization.

Besides the suggestion to actually program generalization, another often-suggested generalization strategy is to "train loosely." This strategy was applied in a study conducted by Campbell and Stremel-Campbell (1982) with two moderately retarded children. The language targets *is* and *are* were taught in a multiple-baseline design across three syntactic structures: *wh-* questions, yes-no questions, and statements. Language training occurred concurrently with academic tasks, such as teaching self-help skills. Generalization probes were conducted within a free-play setting to assess both immediate setting generalization and longer-term maintenance of the language targets. Both children demonstrated spontaneous use of *is* and *are* in the free-play setting, and a trend was evident for maintenance.

STUDIES WITH THE AUTISTIC POPULATION

As many researchers have noted, language generalization has been extremely difficult to achieve with autistic children (Koegel and Rincover, 1974; Lovaas, Koegel, Simmons, and Stevens-Long, 1973). The term "stimulus overselectivity" has been used to describe the characteristic of focusing on one particular aspect of a stimulus complex and "learning" to produce the response only in the presence of that particular aspect. In one study, the table at which training had occurred appeared to be the critical aspect needed to evoke the response—when it was moved to a generalization setting, the trained response was produced. An early study by Lovaas and associates (1973) also revealed the severity of generalization problems in autistic children. Behavioral gains made in treatment were, for all practical purposes, lost in a group of autistic children discharged to an institution, whereas behaviors were maintained or improved in autistic children whose parents were involved in training designed to achieve generalization and maintenance of trained behaviors. With this population especially, attention must be given to factors known to be related to generalization.

The five studies summarized in this section provide a variety of approaches to try when the trained behaviors of autistic individuals are ready to be "encouraged to generalize." Notice the variability within the subject characteristics, as well as the variation in success at achieving some degree of generalization. Table 5–2 indicates the language targets, settings, and results for these studies, which included measures of setting generalization in the autistic population.

Because it has become one of the most frequently cited studies on stimulus generalization and maintenance, the first study described will be the one mentioned previously by Lovaas and co-workers (1973), who reported generalization and follow-up results on multiple-response measures for 13 autistic children subsequent to behavioral treatment. Target behaviors included two behavioral categories that should be decreased if treatment has been effective (self-stimulation and echolalic speech) and three behavioral categories that should increase with treatment (appropriate speech, social nonverbal behavior, and appropriate play). Stimulus generalization was assessed with the children in a nontreatment room, both alone and in the company of an unfamiliar adult—thus, both setting and person generalization data were gathered. During an Attending Condition, the adult attended visually to the child but did not comment or interfere with the child; thus, spontaneous (child-initiated) verbal or social behaviors could be noted. During an Inviting Condition, the adult encouraged the child to participate in activities such as playing "pattycake," answering questions, and obeying commands. Before and after treatment scores averaged over all conditions showed that appropriate behaviors increased and inappropriate behaviors decreased. Interestingly, not until the eighth month of treatment did social nonverbal and self-initiated verbal behavior increase. The investigators noted that language behavior was harder to build than nonverbal social behavior. Individual differences among the 13 children were also noted.

The major finding of the Lovaas and associates study, however, had to do with the follow-up measures that were collected one to four years after termination of treatment. For some of the children, the initial generalization period was an early phase of extinction because the reinforcing contingencies within the nontreatment environments were not sufficient to maintain the positive behaviors. Four children who were discharged to an institution lost gains made in treatment; that is, the learned behaviors were not maintained by contingencies operating in

Table 5–2. Studies of Setting Generalization with the Autistic Population

Authors	Subjects	Output Mode	Language Target	Settings	Results
Lovaas, Koegel, Simmons, and Stevens-Long (1973)	13 children	Speech	Appropriate speech	Training in TR*: probes in nontreatment room; follow-up to institution or homes	4 children discharged to institution lost gains; 9 children discharged to trained parents maintained gains
Rincover and Koegel (1975)	10 children	Motor responses	Receptive understanding of verbal commands, e.g., "Touch your nose" and "Do this"	Training in TR; probes to lawn outside	6 children showed some setting generalization; 4 showed unusual stimulus control
Handleman (1979)	4 boys	Speech	One-word responses to *what* and *where* questions, e.g., "What color is grass?"	Training in both restricted and multiple settings; probes to both	Generalization of answers to home setting; 3 showed higher generalization rates for answers trained in multiple settings
McGee, Krantz, Mason, and McClannahan (1983)	2 adolescents	Choice of obects	Receptive labels for objects used in lunch preparation	Training in kitchen; probes in dining room	Generalization across setting achieved using incidental teaching approach
Carr and Kologinsky (1983)	3 children	Signs	Spontaneous signed requests for foods and activities, e.g., *pretzel, tickle*	Training in 5 different settings; probes to new areas, e.g., art room, school entrance, workshop area	Setting generalization at near-perfect rate for all 3 children

*TR = Treatment room

the natural environment. Self-stimulation and echolalia increased, and social nonverbal behaviors and appropriate verbal and play behaviors decreased. On the other hand, nine children who stayed with their parents maintained gains or improved further. When two of the institutionalized children were reinstated in the treatment program, it was apparent that the children had not "forgotten" the target behaviors—the institutional setting had simply not encouraged them. Thus, children discharged to trained parents tended to improve because they remained in a "treatment environment" that supported the gains made during treatment. The investigators emphasized the heterogeneity of the children, noting that for some children behavioral treatment brought about more change than for others. The stimulus generalization observed was not particularly broad, but this study clearly showed that some setting and person generalization could be achieved with autistic children. Some of the discharged-to-parent children had been treated as inpatients by professionals, whereas others were treated as outpatients, primarily by trained parents, with professionals serving as frequent consultants. Both groups maintained or improved on the follow-up measures.

This study of autistic children points out the importance of preparing the nontreatment environment to support or encourage the language behaviors trained in therapy. Perhaps we could quibble over whether such environmentally supported behaviors deserve to be called "generalized across setting," or "maintained," but the problem is not one of terminology. Unless we as clinicians "cultivate" the natural environment into which we release the language-handicapped child, it is quite likely that some of the behaviors we have labored to establish will fail to thrive in the nontreatment setting. This study will be referred to again in following sections on maintenance and on parent training.

Another often-cited study of autistic children, which raises important concerns about setting generalization for those working with nonautistic children as well, is one by Rincover and Koegel (1975). These investigators assessed the transfer of treatment gains in ten autistic children to the lawn outside the treatment building. Target behaviors included nonverbal imitations in response to "Do this" and a model for some children, and motor responses to verbal commands such as "Touch your nose" for other children. Training in the therapy room consisted of physical prompts, then delay and fading of prompts to transfer control to verbal stimuli, and food and social praise reinforcement. When training criterion was reached, generalization probes (unreinforced) were conducted outside, and one or more correct responses was taken as indicating some degree of transfer. Six of the ten children showed 30 to 80 per cent correct responding, all of them on the first extra-therapy trial (that is, before elimination of reinforcement could be realized). The other four children showed no correct responses, and these are the cases that became famous.

To find out just what aspect of the stimulus complex had been controlling the behavior in the therapy room, these researchers systematically presented various stimuli in the outside setting. For one child, it was a hand-raising movement; for a second child, it was the teacher's letting go of the child's hands; for a third, it was an initial physical prompt; and for a fourth, it was the table and chairs combined with the verbal stimulus. When these stimulus conditions were present in the outside setting, the children's responses transferred, although not 100 per cent correctly. These four autistic children demonstrated unusual stimulus control, in the words of the authors, "...differing considerably from what a typical therapist might expect to occur..." (p. 243).

This study by Rincover and Koegel has been cited subsequently in both the literature on autism and the literature on setting generalization. Although it is an extreme example, perhaps, of the various extraneous attributes of the stimulus complex to which a response can become tied, it should serve to make clinicians aware of just how many stimulus characteristics are potential triggers of the behavior.

In terms of language characteristics of the stimulus, it is important to think of the results of failing to vary the verbal antecedents that evoke the language targets as they are taught. In real-world conversation, verbal antecedents to certain language responses vary considerably. In these cases, the response should *not* become tied to a narrow range of verbal antecedents, such as "Tell me about..." or "What's happening here?" In other cases, such as routine or ritualized greetings and closings, there is a highly predictable sequence of utterances, e.g., "Hi, how are you?"—"I'm fine" or the telephone closing, "O.K., bye."—"Bye." As the target language behaviors become more sophisticated and the cognitive levels of clients more advanced, careful attention must be paid to the verbal antecedents used to evoke desired behaviors in both training and generalization settings.

Several earlier studies had suggested that training in multiple settings could result in some successful setting generalization. This led to an investigation of the generalization effects of training in both restricted and multiple school settings on production of the target behaviors in both restricted and multiple home settings (Handleman, 1979). In a multiple-baseline design across question sets, four autistic boys, who did not use spontaneous language to communicate, were trained to respond with single words to six different sets of questions. These were *what* and *where* questions, such as "What color is grass?" Praise and food were reinforcers in 20 training trials received three times per day within both training settings. Trials were administered by different college-student tutors, with five tutors instructing a child for both restricted and multiple setting conditions. Multiple settings along a mapped route at school included classroom, tutor lounge, coat room, and areas outside bathrooms, by the front door, and by an office. At home, mothers probed for generalization of question-answers in both a restricted setting (kitchen) and along a mapped route that included kitchen, an area outside the bathroom, the child's and parents' bedrooms, and areas near the television and by the front door.

Three of the four boys were similar in their generalization to home probes. Answers were generalized at a higher rate (40 to 80 per cent) for boys trained in multiple school settings than for those trained in restricted school settings (0 to 40 per cent). The fourth boy generalized answers to home probes at a relatively high rate (60 to 100 per cent), regardless of whether training had occurred in restricted or multiple school settings. Response maintenance on subsequent home probes showed relatively high levels for three of the four subjects, but some evidence of extinction for the fourth.

This study was a rather sophisticated attempt to demonstrate that training with both multiple trainers and multiple settings can result in greater generalization of target language responses than can training with one clinician or teacher in only one setting. Unfortunately, the target language behavior was rather artificial. Questions such as "What color is grass?" and "Where do you hang your clothes?" are not common questions that are asked in natural environments. Most natural questions are asked because the asker wants to find out some information—we ask questions because we don't know the answers. Thus, even though this study lets us know that generalization across settings and people (from school to home and from tutors to mothers) is more likely to occur when training occurs in multiple settings, it seems to have included a control *against* the positive influence of programming common stimuli. The clinical implication from this study is to train in multiple settings, but it is possible that the manipulated variables would have had the same effects if more commonly asked questions had been used as the verbal stimuli.

In contrast to the previous study, which neglected to program common stimuli, the study described next used commonly encountered items used in lunch preparation as receptive labels to be learned. This study investigated the teaching and generalization of receptive language targets and used a modified incidental teaching approach with autistic youths who had been institutionalized (McGee, Krantz, Mason, and McClannahan, 1983). In this approach, the natural environment is arranged to attract children to desired objects, materials, and activities, and the teacher provides attention, praise, and instruction when a communicative attempt is made.

Subjects were two adolescent youths who had been transferred from an institution to a group home. Both had basic direction-following skills and limited expressive speech. Four sets of objects used in daily lunch preparation (baggie, lettuce, relish) were taught in a multiple-baseline design across object sets, with replication across the second youth. Each set included three target objects and two distractor objects related to lunch preparation. Training procedures included establishing a "ready" set, requesting an object, giving a gestural prompt when needed, and providing tokens or behavior-specific praise contingent on cooperative participation. When the youth completed a set, he or she could proceed with lunch preparation. A teaching-parent conducted both the training and generalization phases, moving from kitchen to dining room setting to probe for generalization of object labels. Generalization probes were separated from training sessions by at least one intervening activity. As is common in behavioral research, no tokens, praise, or feedback were given during generalization probes.

Results showed increases in correct responding during both teaching and generalization conditions, with percentage correct appearing to be slightly lower for the generalization condition. Incorrect responses were nearly all errors of commission; i.e., subjects gave the teacher some object, though not always the correct one. Generalization across settings and time-of-day was successfully achieved in this study, using a modified incidental teaching approach alone, with no additional technique used to encourage generalization. This study is particularly encouraging and adds support to the notion that training within natural environments, using common stimuli of functional value to the impaired individual, can effect a healthy degree of generalization.

In discussing their application of incidental teaching procedures with autistic children, McGee and co-workers presented several considerations to keep in mind to prevent stimulus overselectivity for the receptive language targets used in their experiment. They also suggested that generalization was facilitated as a result of teaching in the context of activities where naturally occurring events maintain the target behavior—and community-based group home settings seem to be particularly good places to work on generalized language behaviors.

It is one thing to succeed at getting a language-handicapped child to display trained language in new settings or with new people in response to antecedent events that have been learned in therapy. Such verbal antecedents as "Tell me about this" or "What's this?" or "What's happening here?" are used to train a language response, then become the trigger for a display of trained language outside of therapy. It is quite another thing, however, to get the child to display the trained language spontaneously—that is, in response to some internal motivation or an environmental event that would appropriately trigger language in normal speakers.

Such spontaneity of production was the goal of Carr and Kologinsky (1983), after training had successfully established a sign language repertoire in six autistic children. During a 30-session baseline, observation revealed the virtual absence of *spontaneous* signing, even though children had 25- to 50-sign repertoires. The children were taught by imitative prompting, fading, and differential reinforcement procedures, and aspects of incidental teaching were also used in the program. Spontaneity was defined in accordance with the Lovaas and associates (1973) definition; that is, production was considered spontaneous only if the teacher had not prompted or asked questions.

Signs chosen represented ten reinforcer items that could be consumed or played with or reinforcing activities—thus, signed requests were reinforced by the natural consequence of receiving what was requested. Training sessions were daily 5- to 10-minute periods. After the first session, during which imitative prompts were used exclusively, each training session began with the teacher eye-contacting the child and waiting. If after 5 minutes signs for all ten reinforcers had not been displayed, imitative prompting was again used. Gradually, stimulus control was transferred from imitative prompts to the mere presence of an attending adult. A reversal-reinstatement design showed that the intervention procedures increased spontaneous signing and decreased self-stimulatory behavior (Carr and Kologinsky, 1983). Thus, spontaneous signing *can* be taught by systematic application of procedures such as imitative prompting, fading, and differential reinforcement.

A second experiment with three additional subjects replicated the first and also investigated generalization to settings and people. Training was conducted in five different settings, and setting generalization was achieved at nearly perfect rates for all three children. Generalization across adults was investigated using two of the children and was high for one but lower and less stable for the other.

In discussing their study, Carr and Kologinsky (1983) contrasted the roles that two commonly used teaching procedures may play in language teaching—discrete trial teaching and incidental teaching. For teaching *forms*, such as labels, the discrete-trial procedures appear to be quite effective. However, for teaching *use*, the incidental teaching method appears to be quite effective. The two procedures should be viewed as complementary rather than dichotomous, since without the sign repertoire built up by discrete-trial training, it is unlikely that the success in achieving spontaneity of production via incidental teaching tactics would have been achieved.

This study by Carr and Kologinsky provides a good illustration of the combination of several of Stokes and Baer's generalization strategies. Training multiple exemplars (ten different requests and training in five different settings) and programming common stimuli (reinforcer items and attending adults) were used.

STUDIES WITH THE LANGUAGE-IMPAIRED POPULATION

The five studies summarized in this section included young language-delayed, nonretarded children. Measures of setting generalization were collected in home or free-play settings. Table 5–3 indicates the language targets, settings, and results for these studies.

One of the goals for young language-delayed or language-impaired children may be simply to increase the amount of talking, especially in nontreatment settings. It is often the case that children respond to training stimuli during therapy but produce little spontaneous language outside the treatment setting. In an attempt to get children to display the language behaviors taught in therapy sessions during classroom free-play periods, Rogers-Warren and Warren (1980) applied a modified incidental teaching approach. Using a multiple-baseline design across children, these researchers showed how systematic changes in adults' instructions for verbalizations, models for verbalizations (mands), and contingent positive consequences following utterances could double or triple children's verbalization rates from their baseline levels. Teachers prompted language usage and provided the materials, services, or activities requested or described by the children. In addition to increasing the rate of talking, these procedures increased the children's vocabulary and complexity of utterances. Words and grammatical structures taught in therapy were produced by the children in the classroom.

Thus, this study demonstrated that setting and person generalization can be achieved by application of various aspects of an incidental teaching approach. By means of changes in classroom teachers' behaviors—both verbal antecedents and nonverbal consequences—opportunities were provided for children to display the language they were learning in therapy. This would require close interaction and cooperation between speech-language clinicians and classroom teachers and some joint decision-making about the language behaviors to teach.

A study similar to the one above applied the mand-model procedure to three unresponsive language-delayed preschool children in a morning free-play session and assessed generalization of teacher language behavior as well as child language behavior in an afternoon free-play session (Warren, McQuarter and Rogers-Warren, 1984). The child

Table 5–3. Studies of Setting Generalization with the Language-disordered Population

Authors	Subjects	Language Target	Setting	Results
Rogers-Warren and Warren (1980)	3 children	Verbalization rates, words, and grammar	Training in TR*; probes in classroom, free-play setting	Setting generalization to free-play setting
Warren, McQuarter, and Rogers-Warren (1984)	3 preschool children	Obligatory and nonobligatory verbalizations	Training in one free-play setting; probes in second free-play setting	Setting generalization to second free-play setting; rates maintained after teachers reduced mand-model frequency
Hegde (1980)	2 children	*Is* copular and auxiliary in simple sentences	Training in TR; probes in nontreatment room and home settings	Setting and person generalization in conversational speech
Hegde, Noll, and Pecora (1979)	1 child	Contracted copular and auxiliary *'s*, *was*, and possessive *'s*	Training in TR; probes at home	Setting and person generalization on structured probes
Hughes (1982)	4 children	*Is* and *are* as copular and auxiliary in spontaneous language	Training in TR; probes in home	Low rates of setting generalization in conversational speech; generalization failure concluded

*TR = Treatment room

language behaviors targeted were verbalization rates for both obligatory language (responses to non–yes-no questions, instructions to verbalize, and models) and nonobligatory language (requests).

Four teachers in a special preschool were trained in the use of mands and models to prompt child speech and in the use of positive feedback for child verbalizations in obligatory speech situations. Baseline observations of five teacher behaviors in an early free-play setting showed few of the mand-model behaviors. During an initial intervention phase, teachers used the mand-model procedure at least ten times over a 15-minute observation period. For a second intervention phase, teachers added prompts onto mands to indicate that a two-word response was required (e.g., "Tell me what this is and use two words.") A third phase, during which teacher instructions and models were decreased, was also described.

Results indicated that certain teacher behaviors generalized to a later free-play setting and that child verbalization rates increased and were maintained above baseline levels in the free-play setting. MLUs increased during the second and third phases for all three subjects. Interestingly, two of the three subjects' verbalization rates actually continued to increase during the maintenance phase, when teacher instructions and models were faded. During this phase, teachers maintained their overall interaction rate by asking more non–yes-no questions while decreasing instructions and models. Apparently, the intervention procedures affected both teacher and child language behaviors, and both showed some generalization and maintenance effects.

As in many other intervention studies, this one did not report whether or not the children's target language behaviors (increased output and longer MLUs) occurred outside the school setting or with people other than the four teachers. However, if such generalization did not occur, the mand-model procedure could readily be taught to parents or other listeners frequent in the child's natural environment, thus changing the nontreatment setting in the direction of the treatment setting where success had been demonstrated.

Both setting and person generalization measures were included in a study by Hegde (1980) designed to explore grammatical forms as response classes. Two five-year-old language-delayed children who produced no auxiliary or copular forms of *is* in spontaneous speech were trained in a reversal-reinstatement design to produce either the copular or auxiliary form. After approximately two weeks during which the children's sentence productions were trained, reversed, and reinstated, probes of the child's conversational speech were made under three conditions: with the experimenter in the treatment room, with the experimenter, a student clinician, and the child's mother in a nontreatment room, and with parents at home.

Generalization rates of 89 to 93 per cent correct occurrence in obligatory contexts within the conversations were observed. Some of the contexts were evoked by questions like the ones used in training, and this similarity between the auditory-verbal stimuli used in training (*wh*-questions) and in the generalization setting may have cued the child to produce *is* correctly. Thus, while some generalized productions were descriptive sentences unprompted by verbal stimuli, others were responses to practiced questions. Approximately 60 to 70 per cent of the target sentences in the probes were reported to be novel; the remaining sentences had been practiced in the training sessions. Thus, it is unclear how many of the correct *is* sentences were spontaneous in that they were neither prompted by *wh*- questions nor practiced sentences from the training sessions. Still, given the brief period of training, such high levels of generalization to spontaneous production are encouraging.

Generalization probes administered by a parent at home were also used in a study by Hegde, Noll, and Pecora (1979). Two subjects, aged three and four years, were trained to produce grammatical targets, such as contracted copular and auxiliary *'s*, uncontracted copular and auxiliary *was* and *is*, and possessive *'s*. A multiple-baseline design across grammatical targets was used. For one of the subjects, structured probes to measure generalization across setting (home) and person (mother) were administered when each target reached criterion. For these probes, the verbal stimuli used in training and generalization probes were the same, but interspersed trials (alternation of trained and untrained stimuli) were not used for the generalization probes.

Results indicated 100 per cent correct production of the grammatical targets on the home generalization probes, indicating generalization across setting and person. The use of blocks of ten untrained sentences, all unreinforced, apparently did not reduce correct responding. The generalization probes, however, were highly structured, and no information as to whether the grammatical targets were correctly produced in spontaneous conversational speech was provided.

Another study that included probes of children's spontaneous language at home with parents was carried out by Hughes (1982). The study was designed to investigate the relationship between the type of training program (highly structured versus loosely structured) and the rate of generalization of grammar targets to spontaneous production. During a four-week training program, copular *is* was trained via one program and copular *are* was trained via the other program in four language-impaired children. While high levels of within-therapy responding were achieved, little generalization to spontaneous language produced in the child's home was observed. Neither a highly structured nor a loosely structured treatment program was successful in achieving the 80 to 90 per cent generalization rates observed by Hegde (1980). The highest rate of target production within home-gathered language samples occurred for *is*, a 56 per cent correct production rate for one of the four subjects on the final probe. For many of the samples from all subjects, no correct productions were observed, although opportunities to produce the targets were present. The generalization sampling conditions for this study were quite rigorous, in that the children were fitted with FM transmitters that broadcast their speech to a centrally located tape recorder in the house, and any speech to parents or siblings occurring during a 30 to 45-minute period was recorded. Parents did not know what targets were being treated, and they did not ask any specific questions or prompt language in any noticeable way.

The Hegde and Hughes studies, taken together, show the variation that is probably typical among language-disordered children in their rates of generalization from treatment setting to home settings, from clinicians to parents, and from structured productions to spontaneous productions. Perhaps some factors involved in the treatment programs could account for the differences in subjects' generalization rates. Alternatively, the methods of collecting spontaneous language samples may have differed in some crucial way, thus affecting the generalization rates observed. Or perhaps the subjects themselves differed in their capacity to generalize trained language behaviors to spontaneous production.

SUMMARY

The studies presented in this section shed some light on generalization of learned language behaviors across settings. These studies included a good variety of language targets, ranging from receptive understanding of object labels to production of complex *if-then* sentences. Subjects of the studies included profoundly retarded institutionalized adults, autistic adolescents, and language-delayed children. Some of the studies included measures of setting generalization alone, whereas others included measures of generalization across both setting and persons.

Given this heterogeneous sample of research on generalization of language behaviors across settings, general conclusions concerning achievement of setting generalization are not readily drawn. In some cases, generalization across settings may occur with no extra programming needed. In other cases, setting generalization may not occur, and some degree of extra programming will be necessary. Strategies for achieving generalization across settings may include conducting the initial training within multiple settings or implementing training within the generalization settings, once probes have revealed that such generalization has failed to occur. Another variable that may affect the amount of setting generalization observed is the choice of targets; i.e., common, functional language targets seem to be more likely to generalize across settings. The use of multiple trainers, even within a single treatment room, might also facilitate setting generalization, although the experimental studies reviewed have not addressed this possibility in a clean design.

In conclusion, more research is needed to clarify the role of several factors in achieving generalization across settings. The phenomenon is complex and probably interacts with a number of other variables known or suspected to influence generalization of language behaviors, for example, the audiences found in various nontreatment settings. In the following chapter, generalization of language target behaviors across persons or listeners will be explored.

Chapter 6
Stimulus Generalization Across Persons

If one of our prime objectives in treating language-handicapped clients is to help them successfully participate in communicative interactions with other people in their environments, then it is important to work toward achieving generalization across a wide variety of persons. To achieve generalization across persons, those persons to whom we want the language targets to generalize can be brought into the therapy sessions, or we can arrange to treat the clients within settings where several different people can be included in the treatment as listeners. Eventually, we want the language behaviors to occur with people who have not been present during treatment, as long as such interaction is appropriate.

As with programming for generalization across other parameters, it may be efficient to combine several aspects, such as person and setting, rather than to change only one aspect of the stimulus complex at a time. To measure generalization across persons, probes may be structured, consisting of a set of trained or untrained items, or both, administered by a nontrainer, or probes may be unstructured, for example, spontaneous language samples with people not involved in training.

As a straightforward example of successful generalization from a trainer to a nontrainer, consider a study of echolalic children by Schreibman and Carr (1978). Two children, one schizophrenic and one retarded, were trained to respond with "I don't know" rather than echo *wh-* questions. In a multiple-baseline design across subjects, a verbal prompt-fading procedure was used to teach the desired response to a *wh-* question randomly chosen from among a pool of ten *what, how,* and *who* questions, such as "What are we doing?" and "How is your tummy?" Answers to known questions, such as "What's your name?" were included in training to ensure discrimination between questions to be answered by "I don't know" and questions to which a known answer should be given. Figure 6–1 illustrates the decrease in echolalic responses and the increase in "I don't know" responses for the two children. After reaching criterion, a set of untrained *what, how,* and *who* questions was used to probe whether generalization to untrained questions had occurred. After generalization to the untrained *what, how,* and *who*

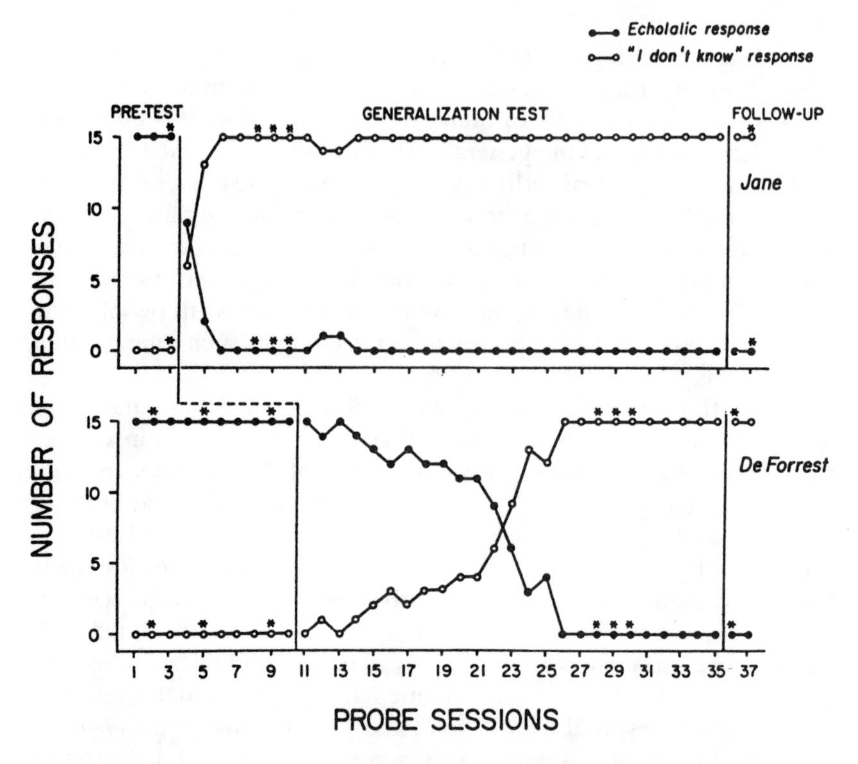

Figure 6–1. Data from a multiple-baseline design across two subjects showing generalization of a target response ("I don't know") to untrained questions and to persons not involved in training (asterisks indicate data collected by naive experimenters). From Schreibman, L., and Carr, E. (1978). Elimination of echolalic responding to questions through the training of a generalized verbal response. *Journal of Applied Behavior Analysis, 11,* 459. Copyright 1978 by the Society for the Experimental Analysis of Behavior, Inc. Reprinted by permission.

questions reached criterion, a set of *where, why,* and *when* questions (e.g., "Why do rabbits run?", "Where do fish swim?") was used to determine generalization to untrained *wh-* words.

For certain probes of both sets of questions, an adult naive about the purpose of the study asked the questions, in order to examine any experimenter-specific effects of training. In Figure 6–1 these probes are indicated by an asterisk. Results of this study revealed response generalization across a broad set of untrained questions, regardless of who asked them. The "I don't know" response generalized from trainer to nontrainer. Follow-up measures one month after termination of treatment indicated that the response was maintained.

A number of the studies described in the previous chapter on stimulus generalization across settings also included stimulus generalization across persons. In the nontreatment setting, a person other than the clinician or trainer administered the generalization probes. If person and setting generalization occur spontaneously, no further programming is required. However, in some cases, the trained language response did not occur in the new setting until the person there carried out some training, that is, applied contingencies to the behavior (Garcia, 1974). However, once this extra treatment had been applied in the first generalization setting, transfer occurred to a second generalization setting without training by the person there. Thus, additional training by a person other than the original trainer in a nontreatment setting may be needed before spontaneous generalization to a third setting and person is observed.

GENERALIZATION FROM TRAINER TO NONTRAINERS

There have been several studies that investigated generalization of language behaviors to people not involved in training (i.e., nontrainers) after a trainer or clinician has established the specific language target. Sometimes generalization is assessed by using only one person not involved in training, whereas for other studies, several persons not involved in training have been used to assess generalization of a particular language skill. In the following sections, generalization studies of language-handicapped subjects from various populations will be described. Note the variety in language targets and in the methods for assessing generalization across persons.

Studies with Language-Disordered Children

Parents of language-delayed or language-disordered children have been recruited to administer structured and spontaneous probes of generalization across persons after a period of treatment has established language targets. Alternatively, mothers have been trained to administer a treatment program at home, and clinicians have assessed generalization across persons. Table 6–1 summarizes several studies of language intervention that have included measures of generalization across persons.

After training on various grammatical targets (e.g., contracted auxiliary and copular *'s, was,* possessive *'s*) had resulted in generalization to untrained sentences on clinic structured probes, generalization to mother at home was assessed for one of the subjects in a study by Hegde, Noll, and Pecora (1979). The child's mother was given stimulus pictures and written questions designed to elicit target sentences on a structured probe at home. Results indicated no problems in generalization of structured responses across person and setting (Hegde et al., 1979).

Conversational parent-child probes have also been used to assess generalization of grammatical targets across persons and settings (Hegde, 1980). Following achievement of criterion on the reinstatement phase of a single-subject reversal design used to investigate formation of a response class, the production of *is* in conversational speech was assessed during sessions in the clinic with the child's mother and at home with both parents. Results indicated that the trained grammatical feature had generalized to conversational production across settings and persons with 89 to 93 per cent accuracy. Thus, for both these studies generalization of grammatical targets across persons was achieved without using the parents during training.

Generalization from clinician to mother following a period of treatment was also reported by Zwitman and Sonderman (1979). Eleven language-delayed preschool children who had been selected on the basis of performance on a delayed imitation pretest were administered a seven-step syntax teaching program, which included daily home practice with the child's mother. Post-treatment data were collected two to six months after pretesting. Mean difference scores were significantly higher for the treated group than for a matched, untreated group.

However, there was considerable variability in the generalization of trained structures to spontaneous speech. Analysis of language samples showed that two of eight children receiving training on auxiliary *is* failed to use this form in conversational speech with their mothers in a clinical setting, even though they had produced the form on the structured post test. When asked to self-correct, the two children were able to do so. Similarly, three of ten children who had been trained on

Table 6–1. Studies of Language-deficient Subjects that Included Measures of Generalization Across Persons

Authors	Subjects	Language Target	Results
Hegde, Noll, and Pecora (1979)	1 language-delayed child	Pronouns, auxiliary verbs, and possessive *'s*	Generalization to mother at home on structured probes
Hegde (1980)	2 language-delayed children	*Is* as copular and auxiliary verbs in sentences	Generalization to mothers in nontreatment clinic room and at home on conversational probes
Zwitman and Sonderman (1979)	11 language-delayed children	Grammar targets, e.g., auxiliary *is,* articles	Most but not all children showed generalization to spontaneous language samples collected by mothers
Mahoney and Snow (1983)	14 preschool Down's syndrome children	Receptive language, imitation, and conversation	Lessons were taught by mothers; performance was assessed by clinician; post-treatment assessment indicated substantial improvement in rate of language acquisition on various measures
Faw, Reid, Schepis, Fitzgerald, and Welty (1981)	6 institutionalized MR adults	Three sets of signs for desired objects or food, e.g., candy, TV	Signs were taught by staff persons in small groups; generalization to a nonstaff person on structured probes, but little generalization to staff-resident interactions at nontraining times
Rychartik and Bornstein (1979)	3 MR adults	Conversational questions and positive conversational feedback	Generalization to unfamiliar conversational partners (college students) during 4-minute conversations; quantitative measures showed improvement but qualitative ratings did not
Senatore, Matson and Kazdin (1982)	35 MR adults	Verbal social skills, e.g., appropriate multiword responses, positive statements, acknowledging others	Generalization to new role-play scenes and to parties where students asked questions and later rated subjects' answers; treatment with active rehearsal was more effective than without; maintenance at 6 months with only minor losses

articles failed to produce these forms in conversational speech, though the forms were produced correctly on the post test. When asked to self-correct, however, these children were unable to do so. Not only do these results cast doubt on the validity of imitation testing as measures of learning for grammatical targets, but they show that individual children vary in their learning patterns.

Results of the Zwitman and Sonderman study are encouraging in that 70 to 78 per cent of the children showed generalization of trained forms to spontaneous production in language samples with their mothers, without specific programming subsequent to treatment. Inclusion of the mothers in the treatment program may have played a role in the generalization to spontaneous production, even though the procedures used by the mothers were rather highly structured. Controlled studies of the effects of various kinds of parent treatment are needed before the relationship between parent teaching and generalization across persons is clear.

Another parent-administered language training study, which used a number of pre- and post-treatment measures of language gains, was carried out with 14 Down's syndrome children ranging in age from 24 to 36 months (Mahoney and Snow, 1983). This study was designed to investigate the relationship between cognitive and sensorimotor functioning and language intervention. Mothers received four weekly sessions of individualized instruction on the teaching procedures used in the *Environmental Language Inventory* (ELI) (MacDonald and Nickols, 1978) during Phase I. Procedures included modeling, shaping, recording behavioral change, and adapting procedures to the child's capabilities.

During the two months of Phase II, weekly visits continued, and mothers began administering daily language lessons designed to teach words and early multiword relational meanings. Children were assessed by the language trainer to determine learning of the previous week's objectives, and new lessons were prepared in accordance with ELI recommendations. Lessons included receptive language training, imitation training, conversation training, a structured play session to elicit items correctly produced in imitation or conversation, and generalization training. Mothers practiced the lesson and were provided feedback regarding their performance. For the next three months (Phase III), mothers assumed primary responsibility for designing and implementing the weekly language lessons, with weekly telephone calls and monthly home visits by the trainer.

Pre-intervention and post-intervention scores were obtained for the *Receptive-Expressive Emergent Language Scale* (REEL) (Bzoch and League, 1971), the *Bayley Scales of Infant Development* (Bayley, 1969), the *Ordinal Scales of Psychological Development* (Uzgiris and Hunt, 1975), the *Environmental Pre-language Battery* (MacDonald and Nichols, 1978), and maternal reports of the number of words their children had produced spontaneously at least three times in appropriate social situations. Results indicated substantial improvement in rate of language acquisition. Of special interest for generalization strategists is the fact that the number of words reported spontaneously produced increased by more than 200 per cent over the course of intervention, although there was considerable variability among children.

Since the Mahoney and Snow study was designed to explore the relationship between cognitive functioning and language learning, the results shed some light on the behaviorist versus developmentalist approaches to language intervention. Briefly, some behaviorist positions often advocate choosing targets based on functional need rather than on developmental sequence and ignoring children's cognitive status (Mahoney and Snow, 1983; Brinker and Bricker, 1979). Developmentalist positions advocate choosing targets based on what is known about normal language development sequences and may assess or even train sensorimotor cognitive skills as part of language intervention (Mahoney and Snow, 1983). Correlations among gain scores and cognitive variables found in the Mahoney and Snow study indicated that children's level of language functioning both before and after intervention were highly correlated with pre-intervention cognitive levels.

However, measures of criterion achievement, such as the verbal and nonverbal scores on the *Environmental Pre-language Battery*, were not systematically related to cognitive functioning. These results are consistent with the behaviorist position that level of cognitive functioning is irrelevant for language acquisition; i.e., children at all levels of cognitive functioning were capable of learning individually defined language objectives. Nevertheless, the measures of language gain that reflected *spontaneous* generalization to the natural environment—e.g., expressive language scores on the REEL and number of words reported—were related to cognitive levels. Mahoney and Snow concluded that "... cognitive status seems to be a critical factor for the generalized use of spontaneous communication" (p. 253). They went on to advocate training on both preverbal communication skills and on sensorimotor skills, as part of early language intervention.

Studies with the Adult Mentally Retarded

The previous studies with language-disordered children often involved parents, especially mothers, as the persons to whom generalization of the language targets was desired. With the population of mentally retarded adults, especially those in institutions, parents may not be the logical persons for assessing and programming generalization. Rather, staff members or other personnel employed in the residential facilities may be the persons to use in assessing and programming generalization of language behaviors. Table 6–1 summarizes several studies which have included generalization across persons.

As a result of earlier work suggesting that involvement of the direct-care staff in institutional settings is crucial to facilitating the use of sign language by residents, a study designed to describe and evaluate methods of involving direct-care personnel in sign language intervention was carried out (Faw, Reid, Schepis, Fitzgerald, and Welty, 1981). Three male and three female staff members were trained to carry out sign teaching to six residents during an evening shift. Group training sessions were conducted four or five days per week for 10 to 15 minutes until three sets of signs were learned. Each set consisted of three signs for objects or food (e.g., *candy, banana, TV*), which were considered by the personnel to be ones that could be used in typical interactions between staff and residents. Two staff persons provided instructions, models, physical guidance, and contingent feedback, praise, and edible treats for correct signing to three residents at a time. The verbal antecedent, "What is the sign for (name of item)?" and a picture of the referent were used to teach each sign individually until all three residents could demonstrate it. Supervisors implemented procedures to maintain the staff's training interactions, providing verbal prompts and positive feedback to the staff. Baseline measures and post-training measures were carried out by a nonstaff person, using the same verbal antecedent used in training, in individual sessions. This allowed for measurement of generalization across persons and from group to individual interaction.

Results of the first experiment, a modified multiple-baseline across sets of signs, showed that correct sign production increased by at least 33 per cent from baseline to post-training for each resident, with a group mean of 63 per cent. Thus, at least some generalization across persons was shown on structured measures of generalization. However, when observations were made in the natural environment, little generalization was noted. During staff-resident interactions at leisure time and supper time, staff signing was observed only 15 per cent of the time, and no changes in resident signing or vocalizing from baseline rates was noticed.

Subsequently, a second experiment, using real objects rather than pictures and structured interactions during generalization measurement, was carried out. Again, a nonstaff person gathered baseline and post-training data in response to the same verbal antecedent used in the first experiment (i.e., "What is the sign for [name of item]?") and presentation of actual objects encountered during walks through the living unit. For the nine signs initially trained via pictures, there was a mean of 49 per cent correct sign production across all residents, with one resident correctly signing all nine signs. Thus, at least some generalization from picture to real object occurred for all six residents. The number of sessions required to meet criterion varied from 1 to 20 for the four additional signs.

Generalization results for this second experiment by Faw and coworkers revealed that residents correctly produced 78 per cent of the signs trained using real objects when post-tested by the nonstaff person. Thus, generalization from staff trainers to a nonstaff person was observed. Furthermore, three follow-up probes carried out 39 to 49 weeks after training had ceased showed maintenance of signs at approximately post-test levels. Thus, residents learned to communicate with staff via sign language during structured interactions, and signing skills were maintained for a lengthy period. Unfortunately, no measures of staff-resident interaction in unstructured situations were reported for the second experiment. Therefore, it is unknown whether signing generalized to spontaneous resident-initiated communication in unstructured situations.

This study illustrates the application of several techniques considered to be facilitators of generalization. Training was done by the staff, i.e., persons frequently encountered in the residents' natural environment. Targets were chosen after consultation with staff and were items that were considered typical in the natural environment. Real objects, rather than pictures, were used in the second experiment. These factors probably enhanced the chances for generalization of the signs.

For clinicians working in or consulting for residential institutions for the adult retarded populations, this study by Faw and co-workers may offer some ideas for procedures to facilitate generalization of language behaviors to persons within these settings. It would be interesting to know whether the residents began signing to each other and to what extent they initiated signing, rather than merely responding to questions and prompts. Perhaps future experimental studies will address these issues.

Higher-functioning mentally retarded adults were taught several conversational skills, and generalization to a number of nontrainers was measured in a study by Rychtarik and Bornstein (1979). In a multiple-baseline design, three behaviors were trained in phases within three subjects: eye contact, conversational questions, and positive conversational feedback. Only one person administered the training. To assess generalization across persons, four 4-minute conversations between the subject and a different unknown conversant were videotaped during each training phase. Conversational partners were 12 female and 3 male undergraduate university students who had received training to make no initiations, limit questions to 15 seconds or less, keep relatively constant eye contact, and limit head nods and acknowledgments to no more than six per conversation. To teach the subjects, a seven-step training sequence was applied for all three behaviors. The sequence included oral instructions, observation of a model videotape, summary of the material, quizzing of subjects to ensure understanding, rehearsal and videotaping of subjects, viewing of the videotape with feedback, and instructions to practice. Results indicated that training increased the frequency of the three conversational behaviors with unknown conversants over baseline levels for all three subjects. For example, the number of conversational questions increased for one subject from a baseline of 2 to 11; for another subject, questions increased from 22 to 31, following initiation of treatment.

Even though quantitative measures showed improvement, more qualitative measures did not. Overall conversational ability ratings by staff members at a workshop for the retarded subjects showed little change along the six-point semantic differential scale after treatment. Thus, despite increases in the target behaviors, improvement in overall conversational abilities was minimal, at least as perceived by the raters.

Nevertheless, this study provides some interesting ideas for treating conversational language skills and a way for mentally retarded adults to practice them with unfamiliar listeners. Specific target behaviors were provided (e.g., "Tell me more about that" or "That's nice") that could be taught to and practiced with adult clients in need of conversational skills. For this study, college students were used to measure generalization to nontrainers. In lieu of such a pool of conversants, adult volunteers might be used as part of the treatment program. Perhaps a community setting for mentally retarded adults has a volunteer program that encourages involvement of students and other interested persons to increase interaction with these individuals. A brief training procedure for instructing volunteers in how to improve conversational skills of the mentally retarded adults may be a viable way to achieve some generalization of language target behaviors.

Attention must also be given to the measurement of such language behaviors as conversational skills. While behavioral programs and experimental research emphasize counting behaviors, increases in frequency do not always mean clinically significant changes. Perhaps more emphasis on developing measurement tools that reflect the lay person's perception of effective communication is needed. In many cases, good verbal communication skills may not show up as simply high frequencies of certain behaviors, but as an appropriate balance between occurrence of the behavior in some contexts and nonoccurrence of it in other contexts.

As a further example of rating scale measurement of the generalization of verbal social skills in mentally retarded adults, a large-group study by Senatore, Matson, and Kazdin (1982) is presented. Thirty-five adults in the borderline to severe range, who could speak in at least four-word sentences, were divided into a control group and two treatment groups. One treatment group received a standard social-skills training package that employed instructions, modeling and role playing of scenes, and social reinforcement, but no active rehearsal. The other group received a similar program, but individuals were required to act out scenes by walking through and overtly rehearsing the situations, with prompts given by the therapist. Sessions of 1 hour were held twice weekly for five weeks in small groups of three to five clients. Attendance and paying attention were reinforced with soft drinks at the end of the session. For both groups, half of the scenes were those used for pre- and post-testing and half were suggested by the clients. Assessments included an audiotaped role-play scene requiring display of social skills (e.g., positive statements, acknowledging others, and complaining) and an audiotaped ten-question interview with two nontrainers. An example of a role-play scene used in assessment was the following:

> You have just come to the hospital for a group meeting. You missed the meeting last week and you are wondering if other group members will want to talk to you this week.
>
> *Role Model Prompt:* Hi. I'm glad you came today. I missed you last week.
>
> *Narrator to Subject:* You say ... (p. 316)

In addition to these pre- and post-treatment measures, treatment effects were assessed in vivo in a naturalistic setting by using two students trained to work three questions into conversations with each client at a party. The scoring system was based on social behaviors that direct-care staff considered important. The five-point scale ranged from a socially undesirable response through appropriate verbal responses of one to four or more words within 3 seconds or less.

Results of the study indicated that the treatment that included active rehearsal was more effective than the one without such rehearsal. Effects were noted for behaviors not directly treated, such as the responses to interview questions (i.e., response generalization). In addition, treatment effects generalized to the naturalistic setting (party) and were maintained at a six-month follow-up assessment with only minor losses.

This study suggests a number of useful tactics for both initial learning and generalization of conversational language behaviors in mentally retarded adults. Successful generalization to several people not involved in the treatment was demonstrated following five weeks of treatment. Aspects of treatment that were probably conducive to generalization were the small group sessions, which allowed for practice with several different listeners, the choice of functional language targets, use of multiple examples, and application of natural consequences for the target language behaviors. The specific procedures described in this study also suggest that active rehearsal during role playing is more effective than modeling responses and providing feedback. Thus, the results of the Senatore and associates study nicely illustrate a number of the tactics that have been suggested for increasing generalization.

GENERALIZATION EFFECTS OF PEER TRAINING

Several experimental studies have indicated that training peers can result in increases in the language and social behaviors of some populations of language-disordered children (Table 6–2). However, generalization of such effects has been disappointing. Neither the trained behaviors of the peer nor the improved behaviors of the subjects generalize readily. Rather, specific treatment programs seem to be necessary to achieve the desired generalization.

Efforts to investigate the effects of training peers as treatment agents for impaired children began after several studies showed disappointing results in achieving generalization beyond treatment conditions when treatment was adult-mediated. In addition, there was some evidence that adult consequating behaviors served to *terminate* ongoing interaction rather than facilitate it. While intervention increased the frequency of certain social behaviors, the overall effect was to produce brief social exchanges that bore little resemblance to normal interaction patterns (Strain, 1980).

Early observational and intervention research showed that children can exert a powerful influence on each other's social behavior. When two four-year-old age peers were trained to initiate social behavior by saying such things as "Come play" or "Let's play school," the responses of six severely handicapped preschool boys increased while the treatment was in effect. In addition, the *initiations* of positive social behaviors of five of the six subjects increased (Strain, Shores, and Timm, 1977). Since this study did not include generalization measures, a replication was carried out to investigate generalization of treatment effects (Strain, 1977). One age peer was trained to initiate social play with three preschool behaviorally handicapped and retarded children, and generalization to a free-play period in the classroom, with the peer trainer absent, was measured both immediately after the intervention sessions

Table 6–2. Studies that Have Employed Peer Training as Part of Treatment

Authors	Subjects	Target Bahavior	Results
Strain, Shores, and Timm (1977)	6 severely handicapped children	Social responses and initiations	While two trained peers applied treatment (initiating social behavior), responding increased, and for five subjects, initiations also increased; no measure of generalization
Strain (1977)	3 preschool MR children	Positive social responses	For two of three subjects, positive social responses generalized to two free-play periods with the peer trainer absent
Strain, Kerr, and Ragland (1979)	4 autistic children	Vocal-verbal and motor-gestural positive social behaviors	Positive social behaviors increased while peer trainer was present, but not when trainer was absent
Hendrickson, Strain, Tremblay, and Shores (1982)	3 withdrawn preschool children	Vocal-verbal and motor-gestural positive social behaviors	Substantial increases in positive social behavior during treatment sessions, but no generalization by either peer trainer or subjects in a nontreatment play area until peer was prompted and praised for using the trained initiation behaviors
	3 school-age behaviorally handicapped children	(same)	A behaviorally handicapped peer served as trainer; results similar to those above

and 23 hours later. For two of the three subjects, positive social responses occurred at twice the baseline levels in the generalization sessions at both times. Thus, some generalization from peer trainer to other children and to another time period was observed for the subjects in this study. Apparently, the peer trainer did not need to be present for improved social behavior to occur.

Peer training has included both social initiation procedures and prompting and reinforcement procedures. These two procedures were compared as interventions for increasing the positive social behaviors (both vocal-verbal and motor-gestural) of four 9- and 10-year-old autistic children in a withdrawal of treatment design (Strain, Kerr, and Ragland, 1979). A peer trainer was taught to initiate social play by using verbal signals, such as "Let's play blocks" or "Come play," for one treatment. For the second treatment, the peer trainer was taught to prompt the autistic children with directives such as "Roll the ball to ________" or "Say hello to ________" and to reinforce them by using such phrases as "That's the way to play" or "Very nice, ________." After the peer had learned the two treatment procedures, he was instructed not to apply the treatments during baseline sessions and to apply the designated treatment during the two intervention periods. Two subjects were exposed to the prompting-reinforcement treatment first, and two subjects were exposed to the social initiation treatment first. Generalization was measured in the same play room where treatment occurred, but the peer trainer was not present. Thus, the experiment was designed to reveal whether either treatment procedure resulted in increased social behaviors when the person applying the treatment (i.e., the peer) was not available—a rather rigorous measure of generalization across persons.

Results of the study indicated that both intervention procedures were similar in achieving a rapid and dramatic increase in positive social behaviors for all four autistic children during the sessions when the peer trainer applied the procedures. However, unlike results of the earlier study reported by Strain (1977), neither procedure resulted in increased levels of positive social behaviors during the generalization sessions, when the peer trainer was absent (Strain et al., 1979). The investigators concluded that intervention must be implemented across time and settings if generalized social behavior change is to be achieved with autistic children.

A subsequent study of peer training with withdrawn preschool children supported the need for specific generalization programming. In the first of two experiments, a normally functioning preschool child was trained in specific social initiation behaviors, and in a second experiment a behaviorally handicapped peer was similarly trained (Hendrickson, Strain, Tremblay, and Shores, 1982). Three effective social initiation behaviors identified in an earlier study with normal preschool children (Tremblay, Strain, Hendrickson, and Shores, 1981) were taught to the peer trainers. These were play organizers ("Let's play house"), shares (exchange of ball, blocks, cars), and assists (helping a child with or onto a toy). Data collected included these three behaviors and other vocal-verbal and motor-gestural behaviors produced as either initiated or responded behaviors by any child. During the 15-minute intervention sessions, the peer-trainer was prompted and praised for trying to get a specific subject to play with her for a five-minute period, after which she would do the same with a second, then a third subject. Using a withdrawal of treatment design, data were collected for two baseline phases and two intervention phases. A generalization measure was obtained by instructing the peer-trainer and the three subjects to play together in another play area 10 minutes after the intervention session. Thus, generalization of both peer-trainer behaviors and subject behaviors was assessed across setting and time.

Results of this experiment, like those of earlier ones, indicated immediate and substantial increases in positive social behavior during the intervention sessions. However, no positive behaviors by the socially withdrawn subjects were observed in the generalization sessions for the first five days of measurement. Therefore, the investigators decided to initiate the peer intervention during the generalization sessions. The peer-trainer was prompted and praised for using the trained initiation behaviors, turning the generalization session into a treatment session. The same sudden increase in initiations and interactions observed during the intervention phases resulted. Thus, after generalization failed to occur, treatment was begun within the generalization setting.

The second experiment by Henrickson and colleagues replicated the results of the first, using a behaviorally handicapped peer as the trainer and older, more severely handicapped children as subjects. Again, when it was clear that no clinically significant generalization from treatment to generalization sessions would occur, the peer-trainer was instructed to initiate intervention procedures in the generalization setting, with effective results. In comparison with the first experiment, the handicapped peer required approximately twice as much training, direct prompting, and social praise to carry out the intervention procedures as did the normal peer. The investigators pointed out that educational settings with only other withdrawn, handicapped youngsters present will not provide the social stimuli needed to set the occasion for positive social behavior. Indeed, even with trained peers present, little generalization of the social initiation behaviors occurred. If the movement toward mainstreaming is to be effective, it will be necessary to provide systematic instruction and consequences for normally functioning or less handicapped peers in order to achieve generalization of desired social behaviors.

These studies of peer-mediated treatment for social behaviors (which include expressive and receptive language) are disappointing in terms of generalization. They indicate that prompts and consequences may be necessary in all settings to get peers to maintain their trained behaviors, which in turn are necessary to elicit the positive social behaviors from the impaired subjects. This is *not* generalization, according to Stokes and Baer's definition, which requires occurrence of the relevant behavior "... without the scheduling of the same events ... as had been scheduled in the training conditions." It is simply adding treatment to the "generalization" setting.

APPROPRIATE LANGUAGE GENERALIZATION TO STRANGERS

As mentally retarded and autistic adolescents and adults have been transferred out of institutions and into group homes within the community, it has become imperative to address the language behaviors of these clients in terms of appropriate interaction with strangers or persons not encountered daily. Just as normal children may be directly taught not to talk to strangers but to recognize appropriate people in the community to address, the previously institutionalized clients may require direct teaching both for recognizing the circumstances for talking and for using appropriate verbal interaction skills in those circumstances.

It may be helpful to think about some classes of people in various occupations that are frequently encountered throughout a typical week or month. Clerks in grocery stores and department stores may constitute a class of people for whom various questions and responses are appropriate. Consider some standard routines: "May I help you?" "No thanks, I'm just looking" or "I'm looking for paper—where could I find it?" These may be the kinds of functional language behaviors that should be targeted for individuals who will be expected to function independently in the community.

Another class of people might be bus drivers and other transportation workers. Language targets for clients who must arrange their own transportation might include telephoning skills for requesting information about departure times and places and communication routines for interacting directly with people in charge of vehicles. Polite ways to ask for help from fellow passengers may also be an important language behavior to teach.

People in authority—the police, people at an information desk, nurses, doctors, receptionists—may form a class of people who may be approached in an emergency for help. Practice in communicating problems and requests for help should be considered as language targets. A few essential functional communication behaviors, sometimes referred to as survival language, should be taught and practiced in appropriate situations. These should include responses such as names of house parents, address and telephone number for residence, or written versions of this information.

Role-playing, with props to identify people in various community roles, can be used to teach appropriate communication skills across persons. Such role-playing, with instructions, modeling, and rehearsal, was used successfully in the Senatore and associates (1982) study described earlier. Videotapes for feedback on positive and negative verbal and nonverbal behaviors may also be an effective strategy. If possible, using actual people in the treatment sessions would be a good initial step, with the use of actual people outside of treatment performing their community roles being the ideal final step in achieving the desired generalization across persons in various natural environments.

The peer-training strategy discussed in the previous section could be a valuable one for teaching appropriate language behaviors to use in communicating with people in community-living roles. If volunteers are available or can be recruited from high schools or community organizations, they can be taught to prompt, model, and reinforce appropriate language use as they accompany clients on daily living tasks. Portable tape recorders may prove valuable for teaching self-monitoring of some language targets and also for training the volunteers in prompting, modeling, and reinforcement teaching tactics.

GROUP VERSUS INDIVIDUAL TREATMENT

In the university practica of most speech-language clinicians, clients were assigned to a clinician on an individual basis. Many of the intervention procedures were learned and practiced in one-to-one therapy sessions. Occasionally, a few clients may have been grouped, but probably much of the initial clinical intervention took place in individual clinician-client interaction. The one-to-one format has been advocated as the most appropriate arrangement, especially for young or severely handicapped children, because each child displays individual strengths and weaknesses and perhaps attention deficits or disruptive behaviors.

In some cases, and particularly for initial therapy sessions, these may be valid reasons to use individual treatment.

However, when speech-language clinicians graduated and began to work, especially in the public schools where caseloads are high, group therapy sessions became more commonplace. It was simply more efficient to treat children in groups than in one-to-one sessions. Even though clinicians might believe that children would progress faster if individual sessions could be made available with the same frequency as group sessions, real-world conditions dictate the expedient solution of group treatment. Recently, some clinical research has supported the option of group treatment on grounds of *both* efficiency and effectiveness (McCormick and Schiefelbusch, 1984). Group training can be more efficient in terms of both client time and teacher time. In some cases, group instruction resulted in faster learning than one-to-one instruction.

In addition to faster learning (efficiency), language learning may also be evaluated by the degree of generalization that occurs after a language target has been acquired. It seems that learning in small groups may be conducive to such generalization (Oliver and Scott, 1981). A receptive language task, comprehension of the adjectives *hard* and *heavy,* was taught to eight mentally retarded adults, each adjective in either individual or group therapy. Each subject was trained to identify eight hard and eight heavy objects when each was presented with two distractor items, using a seven-step program. All eight target objects were presented during a session, teaching multiple exemplars simultaneously. Praise and candy reinforcers followed correct responses, and incorrect responses were consequated with "No," repetition of the cue, physical guidance for the correct response, then mild social praise. In group sessions of four students, the same steps and procedures were used. In addition, students were asked to watch while other group members were trained. Two generalization probes of untrained hard and heavy objects were conducted, one immediately after subjects reached criterion and the other one week later.

Results of this study indicated that the rate of acquisition, as measured by the number of trials needed to reach criterion, was the same for individual and group treatment. However, on generalization probes using untrained examples, group treatment resulted in significantly greater generalization. Six of the seven subjects who reached criterion correctly identified more untrained objects after group treatment than individual treatment. Generalization was 45 per cent greater when examples of each concept were taught during group treatment.

In discussing their results, Oliver and Scott suggested that the opportunity for observational learning was greater during group treatment.

If each trial by another person were comparable to direct teaching, then each student was exposed to four times as much teaching as would be available in individual sessions. This may have resulted in overlearning, an important variable in transfer of training to novel stimuli.

As the Oliver and Scott (1981) study indicates, group treatment may be a facilitator of generalization. The use of multiple examples, trained simultaneously, may also have been conducive to generalization, but this occurred for both group and individual treatment and thus should have increased generalization for both conditions. Like many other language treatment studies, this one did not include measures of generalization to the natural environment. The task itself is not likely to occur in natural environments, although situations where comprehension of *hard* or *heavy* would be needed could be simulated. Use of candy and praise as reinforcers on a continuous schedule would work against generalization to natural environments; thus, it is likely that additional programming would be needed to achieve generalization to natural environments. Nevertheless, this study provides support for the effectiveness of group treatment in promoting generalization to untrained examples.

Another argument for group treatment is directly related to achievement of generalization across persons. The importance of the individual versus group treatment issue for language intervention is this: Which format is more likely to facilitate generalization? Consider the conditions under which much conversational use of language occurs. Although short exchanges may be frequent as we interact with strangers in dyads, many of our conversations include three or more people. Thus, group treatment may be more similar to many natural environments. In addition, the availability of several different dialogue partners is also a good arrangement for facilitating person generalization for dialogues. Thus, on two counts, group treatment may be considered advantageous for facilitating generalization. Not only are more conversational partners available for practicing dialogue exchanges, but small-group discussions are also possible within group treatment to practice multiperson exchanges.

Whenever one-to-one treatment is used to teach skills such as attending, imitation, and communicative interaction, there are likely to be problems in getting those behaviors to transfer to classrooms. The clinician must be ready with additional programming to achieve generalization of the trained behaviors in group settings, whether these are regular or special education classrooms. Sometimes peer-training can be effective. Classroom teachers can also be agents of generalization by delivering verbal or visual stimuli and thus providing opportunities to respond and by reinforcing particular behaviors. Other alternatives are to teach self-monitoring skills and to provide a reminder to mediate the response in the group setting.

SUMMARY

Generalization across persons can often be programmed simultaneously with generalization across settings. School and home settings naturally include different people. Thus, tactics for achieving generalization across persons may include parents and siblings. Several studies, in addition to those in this chapter, that have included mothers in language treatment programs are described in Chapter 8. Therapy room and classroom probably include different people, although these two settings may often include some persons in common and thus a "bridge" between the two settings. Involving classroom or resource room teachers may be an effective tactic for promoting generalization across persons. Bringing peers into the therapy sessions may be a good strategy to implement for achieving generalization, since the peer may serve as a mediator for the target behavior. Presence of the peer may prompt the language target, and peers may provide natural consequences for reinforcing or maintaining the target.

In summary, after treatment has established a useful language behavior, generalization across several persons must be assessed. If such generalization does not occur, steps must be taken to involve some of those other people in the treatment program. Some may agree to participate in the treatment setting. For others, involvement may consist of providing opportunities and antecedent events for the language behavior, and providing appropriate consequent events within the natural environment. Since language is primarily a tool for communicating with other people, generalization of language targets across a wide variety of persons is a crucial part of a successful intervention program.

Chapter 7

Maintenance of Generalized Language Behaviors

In the literature available on generalization of language as well as other behaviors established during a treatment program, the terms *generalization, maintenance,* and *transfer of training* are often covered within the same section (Kazdin, 1980; Lovaas, 1981; Mowrer, 1977). Certainly, there are important similarities among these concepts and also similar problems in defining them precisely.

According to Hegde (1985), however, the final goal of clinical intervention should not be generalization, but response maintenance in the natural environment. Rather than trying to achieve generalization, conceptualized as behaviors produced in the absence of reinforcement, clinicians should focus on the problems involved in contingency management within nonclinical environments. Instead of trying to get language behaviors to generalize across various parameters and over time when no reinforcers are delivered, this notion of maintenance acknowledges that some kind of contingencies are necessary to maintain behavior. Those interested in maintenance, then, should arrange for natural contingencies found in nontreatment environments to serve as maintaining contingencies for target behaviors.

Many of the recommendations for achieving generalization are identical to those for achieving maintenance. Egel (1981) noted that although separation of generalization and maintenance is empirically possible, the procedures used to promote them are not mutually exclusive. A comparison of Baer's (1981) *How to Plan for Generalization* and Kazdin and Esveldt-Dawson's (1981) *How to Maintain Behavior* shows many similarities. In this chapter several different interpretations of maintenance will be presented, and results of studies that have included measures of maintenance of language behaviors will be summarized. There seems to be no generally agreed-upon specific definition of maintenance. Rather, various investigators have defined and measured maintenance in individual ways.

MAINTENANCE DEFINED

Maintenance, or durability of responding, was defined earlier in this book as generalization over time. Like other kinds of generalization, it is assumed that direct treatment of the behavior must have ceased for true maintenance to be claimed. However, as the term *programmed maintenance* implies, maintenance may also include durable behavior changes when some deliberate changes in nontreatment environments serve to maintain trained behaviors.

A number of aspects of the maintenance concept require further discussion and definition. One of the first issues is what constitutes "time." How much time must elapse between treatment and the maintenance measure? This leads to a second problem concerning the relationship between generalization (across various parameters) and maintenance. Should measures of generalization, which must by definition occur after some period of treatment, be considered maintenance measures also? Or should generalization and maintenance measures be kept distinct?

A second term whose definition is elusive is *treatment*. Suppose we say that generalization or maintenance should refer only to target behaviors produced in the absence of treatment. If, after noting generalization failure, we then apply strategies for achieving generalization or maintenance, do these strategies constitute treatment? If so, measures taken while these strategies are in effect cannot reflect generalization or maintenance. If by treatment we mean some manipulation of antecedent events and delivery of consequent events—even "naturally occurring" ones on a thin, intermittent schedule—then generalization or maintenance strategies do in fact constitute treatment. When, then, can we say that treatment has been terminated, or withdrawn?

A third problem in defining maintenance is measurement. Can maintenance be claimed, or not claimed, if only one follow-up measure is collected? Just as a repeated baseline measure is required to determine whether pretreatment performance shows a rising, falling, or stable trend, a rigorous measure of maintenance should be repeated several times to determine stability. Success or failure of maintenance should not be claimed unless several measures over time are collected.

As was discussed in Chapter 2, the kind of language behavior chosen can affect decisions on how best to measure it. How often should the behavior occur within a given period of time? Does absence of the behavior indicate no maintenance? Not necessarily—only if appropriate occasions to display it occurred and the behavior was not produced.

Does Generalization Include Maintenance or Does Maintenance Include Generalization?

In a global sense, maintenance is shown when any behavior learned in one time period is exhibited again at later times. Since those later times may include conditions similar or dissimilar to those under which the behavior was learned, measures of maintenance may or may not include generalization across parameters such as persons or settings.

For example, a behavior learned in therapy, such as verbal responding to a set of pictures presented by the clinician, may continue at criterion levels when assessed once a month, even though the verbal responses are no longer practiced in therapy. Generalization assessment of those responses may show no transfer across persons, settings, or other similar pictures. In this case, the behavior is showing maintenance but not generalization. On the other hand, after a behavior such as verbal requesting is learned in therapy, it may be observed with nonclinicians, in nontherapy settings, or for untrained objects, when assessed by repeated monthly probes. In this case, both generalization and maintenance of the desired behavior have been shown.

The relationship between generalization and maintenance requires further definition of what kinds of generalization and maintenance are under discussion. It may be argued that generalization across several parameters should be necessary before maintenance can be expected (Warren et al., 1980) or even measured. In this case we are referring to a rather rigorous definition of maintenance, one that requires generalized performance of the behavior outside the treatment setting within many natural environments, after treatment on the behavior has been terminated.

In Figure 7–1 a number of different subtypes of maintenance are illustrated, as shown by branches that describe various conditions of measurement. According to this diagram, the language behavior must be generalized across some parameter, e.g., across several linguistic contexts, before any maintenance measure is appropriate. After that, maintenance may be measured by either structured probes or spontaneous probes across a number of parameters (e.g., persons and settings). The most rigorous measure of maintenance would be that represented by branch 3j, where the generalized behavior is unobtrusively observed as the client interacts with nontrained persons in a setting unchanged by any treatment programming. Less rigorous measures of maintenance are represented by the remaining branches, which involve some stimulus that may trigger the target behavior, e.g., a verbal prompt during the structured probe, a trained person, or an altered setting. Notice

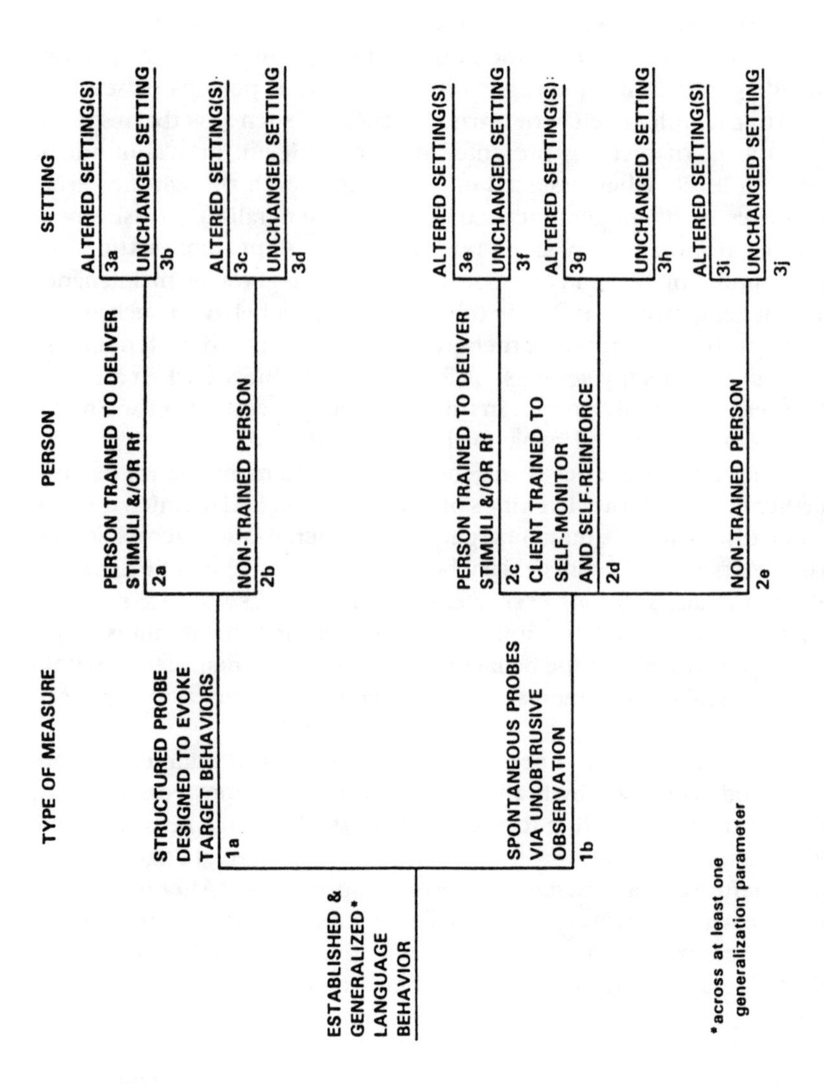

Figure 7–1. Maintenance subtypes, measured after treatment contingencies are withdrawn.

that for all measures of maintenance, *treatment* contingencies have been withdrawn.

It may also be argued, however, that short-term maintenance of the behavior *within* the treatment context might be necessary before generalization can be expected. Indeed, when we include requirements such as "for three consecutive sessions" in our criterion measures, we are addressing the issue of maintenance within the therapy setting. Perhaps it would be useful to distinguish between maintenance of a behavior no longer under treatment, measured within a treatment context, and maintenance of a behavior outside of treatment after all therapy has ceased.

Generalization Over Time: How Long?

The periods across which generalization of a desired behavior may be measured may be short, e.g., several hours, or long, e.g., more than a year. For example, short-term maintenance is shown when a language behavior taught during a morning free-play period is shown during an afternoon free-play period. If short time frames are included in the term *maintenance*, then most of the measures of generalization across parameters such as settings or persons also constitute measures of generalization over time. However, this is not what we generally think of as maintenance.

More often, maintenance implies a rather lengthy period of time between the achievement of a language behavior in treatment and follow-up measures of that behavior one, three, six, even 12 months later. A general rule might be at least two weeks after treatment. Some studies have included maintenance measures as long as a year and a half after direct treatment on the behavior has ended. For example, after intelligible verbal behavior had been increased by delivery of food and praise in two withdrawn chronic schizophrenic patients, assessment a year later showed that levels of verbal behavior close to those achieved in treatment were maintained, even though treatment contingencies had been eliminated (Thompson, Fraser, and McDougall, 1976).

EXPLANATIONS FOR RESPONSE MAINTENANCE

Exactly why responses may be maintained after treatment consequences have been withdrawn is usually not clear (Kazdin, 1980). Although we may speculate that something that was paired with the reinforcer used during treatment may be present in natural environments and continues to act as a reinforcer, this is often difficult to demonstrate. Perhaps some "natural reinforcer" present in nontreatment environments acts to maintain the target behavior.

The notion of "behavioral traps" has been suggested by Baer and his colleagues as such an explanation for maintenance of trained responses (Stokes and Baer, 1977). Such "traps" maintain a behavior that has reached a level sufficient to become "trapped" into a system of reinforcers available in nontreatment environments. Another possibility for explaining maintenance that occurs without additional programming is some permanent change in the agents who administer contingencies during treatment and who continue to be present in the client's environment after treatment has ceased. Although available evidence does not support this explanation, it may be that in some cases, adults in the child's environment may become more systematic in their application of consequences for the target behavior (reinforcement or punishment, or both) after a treatment program has ended. Likewise, adults within the child's environment may offer more opportunities for the desired response to occur after a treatment program has included such a strategy as part of a generalization or maintenance phase. As an example, consider parents who both provide increased opportunities for a language target to occur and follow up with feedback concerning the target several months after treatment has ended.

Both antecedent events that serve to set the occasion for production of the language behavior and consequent events that follow correct and incorrect productions must be considered in explaining maintenance. Since some contingencies must be operating in order for a behavior to be maintained, perhaps an appropriate distinction to make between treatment and maintenance is the artificiality of the contingencies. Within treatment, contingencies for both correct and incorrect productions are artificial, in the sense that they probably would not occur within the natural environment. The same could be said for the antecedent events within treatment. Thus, as the trained behaviors move out of treatment and into natural environments, the kinds of antecedent events and contingencies for the language target behavior change.

Another possibility should be considered as a natural maintaining contingency, and that is the *avoidance* of some negative consequence. Think for a moment about why we do some of the things we do. Perhaps some of our behavior is maintained because we wish to avoid consequences like guilt or low self-esteem. In the case of language behaviors, if parental corrections of an error outside treatment constitute negative consequences, perhaps the child will maintain correct production to avoid them. On the other hand, such corrections may function as reinforcing attention and thus maintain the errored production.

There are many possible consequences of language behavior that might function to maintain various language behaviors in natural environments, and such consequences may be difficult to determine. We may be confident only in saying that they are *not* like the artificial, contrived consequences often used in treatment. Maintenance, then, should not be thought of as occurrence of the trained behaviors in the *absence* of treatment (artificial antecedent events and contingencies) but as occurrence of the trained behaviors in the presence of nonartificial (natural) antecedent events and contingencies.

MEASUREMENT OF MAINTENANCE

For clinicians working in public schools, the measurement of maintenance may be necessary at two levels. At one level, within-treatment measures of previous language targets must be done to check for maintenance. As some of a child's language errors are corrected, periodic checks on these established and generalized behaviors must be made to ensure that they are maintained over time, while therapy continues on additional language targets.

At a second level, maintenance probes must be made of a number of established and generalized targets after a child has been dismissed from treatment, that is, after treatment on all targets has been terminated. These two levels of maintenance might be labeled *within-therapy probes of past targets* and *post-therapy maintenance probes*. Ideally, such post-treatment measures of maintenance would be carried out by nonclinicians or perhaps by a clinician other than the one who treated the client. Thus, generalization across persons would be checked along with maintenance of target behaviors.

TWO KINDS OF MAINTENANCE

Maintenance may occur under both planned and unplanned conditions. Maintenance may sometimes occur automatically following treatment, with no special planning required to achieve it. When this happens, it seems probable that some kind of natural maintaining contingencies are at work. More often, maintenance, like other kinds of generalization, must be planned or programmed as part of a treatment package.

Unplanned Maintenance

When we try to consider what natural maintaining contingencies may take over a language target behavior in the client's natural environment(s) once it has been established by a language treatment program, we may think of both specific and general reinforcers. As an example of specific reinforcers, consider requesting behavior—either verbal or signed. If the target behavior is verbal or signed requests, compliance with such requests for information or objects would constitute a natural reinforcer. When listeners in natural environments grant requests, that requesting behavior should be maintained. Thus, choosing behaviors that others are likely to reinforce should build in natural maintaining contingencies.

Choosing interesting and desirable objects and activities to teach as first words or signs would be another example of planning treatment so that natural contingencies may "automatically" maintain the behavior in nontreatment environments. Intrinsically interesting objects and activities are self-reinforcing, and thus reinforcement should continue after treatment to establish requests for them has stopped.

It may be easy to think of natural reinforcers for requesting behaviors, but what about language that does not request anything? What about speech-act categories such as commenting on events, informing listeners, narrating a story, or using imaginative talk during pretend play? What could be natural reinforcers for such language target behaviors?

As an example of a more general reinforcer of language behavior, consider listener attention. It is highly probable that many of the target language behaviors that are treated will be maintained by listener attention, a powerful reinforcer of language production. For example, once the grammatically correct production of sentences with *is* or *are* or various pronoun targets in the treatment situation have been established and these targets have been found to have generalized across linguistic contexts, persons, and settings, it seems probable that they will be maintained by listener attention whenever they are spontaneously produced in numerous natural environments encountered.

However, it is possible that the same natural reinforcers—listener attention and compliance with requests—previously served to maintain the *errored* language production. Consider a language-delayed child before language treatment has focussed on grammatical features. When the child says, "That not a big one. Me want big piece," chances are that the child receives the listener's attention, the requested item, and perhaps also a verbal acknowledgment. After a period of therapy has established and generalized correct production of the grammar targets, the child may say "That's not a big one. I want a big piece," with the same consequences as before treatment.

It seems rather puzzling that the same natural contingencies can serve to reinforce both incorrect and correct language responses. Nevertheless, it has been noted that during the normal language acquisition process, parents rarely correct grammar errors, but rather respond to the semantic content, accuracy, or truthfulness of the child's utterance. Thus, listener attention probably serves to reinforce both correct and incorrect grammatical productions from normal language learners as well as from non-normal language learners in nontreatment environments. What must happen as a result of treatment is that production of the target must reach a level sufficient for natural reinforcers such as listener attention and compliance to maintain those desired target behaviors.

Planned Maintenance

When maintenance of the language target does not occur automatically, a planned program of treatment is necessary. As was the case with defining generalization earlier, a definition of maintenance must wrestle with what to call the situation in which a behavior is maintained in an altered nontreatment environment.

If the clinician has been successful in implementing the generalization strategy of altering the natural environment, perhaps by increasing the frequency with which important individuals in that environment interact with the client, then the target behavior may be maintained because of this alteration in the natural environment. The increased interaction may provide increased listener attention, a probable natural reinforcer of language. Does this constitute some kind of treatment program? Or consider a more obvious example, where the clinician has succeeded in getting a bus driver, a parent, an older sibling, and a classroom teacher to provide both prompts and praise for a certain language target. If the language target is maintained and generalized, it would be due to programmed maintenance. Perhaps the praise could be faded and the prompts made more subtle with time, and then maintenance of the target would be more similar to the concept of "maintenance in the absence of treatment."

As another example, perhaps a thin schedule of reinforcement consisting of monthly trips contingent on reports of appropriate verbal requests or conversational interaction has been implemented in a sheltered living environment. This may be clearly viewed as treatment, since a contingency is being applied, and thus response maintenance in this situation could not be considered true maintenance either. Perhaps we should look at the varieties of maintenance as occurring along a continuum from highly programmed to more loosely programmed to maintenance in the absence of artificial antecedent events and contingencies. Figure 7–2 illustrates a possible continuum of varieties of maintenance.

A CONTINUUM OF LANGUAGE BEHAVIOR TARGETS

Another factor that may affect maintenance of language behaviors is the kind of language target chosen. Some kinds of language behaviors may require some degree of self-monitoring and reminders to be produced or not produced: consider polite forms or swear words. It may be that the language targets one teaches fall somewhere along a continuum, with automatic, nearly unconscious behaviors at one end and more deliberate, conscious behaviors at the other.

For example, producing grammatical sentences, once grammatical rules are learned, becomes automatic for most speakers. Sentence structure is generally correct regardless of topic, place, listener, or reason for talking. Normal speakers do not seem to consciously arrange the words in sentences according to known grammatical rules. Indeed, speakers often cannot say what the grammar rules are.

Near the other end of the continuum are language behaviors such as greetings and terminations and polite forms such as *please* and *thank you*, which may need to be deliberately produced, at least until they become habitual. Even then, we may consciously choose *not* to greet someone for various reasons. These kinds of language behaviors seem to be more deliberately taught to children, with prompts such as "What do you say to the nice man?" These are not strictly necessary to communicate messages but are necessary if speakers are to be judged communicatively competent in social situations. At this other end of the continuum also are rehearsed speeches, which may require a great deal of conscious planning and deliberate practice to get the words and phrases to come out in desired ways. Certainly, any of these more consciously controlled language behaviors can move toward the less conscious end of the continuum as they are practiced, self-monitored, and reinforced.

In some sense, then, the language behaviors chosen for language-disordered clients may vary in the degree to which they will become automatic, and this may affect the kind of maintenance to expect. Maintenance for language behaviors at the more automatic end of the continuum should eventually reach the stage where no specific maintaining contingencies for them can be determined. Maintenance for language behaviors at the more deliberate end of the continuum may require self-monitoring and self-reinforcement programs to be maintained.

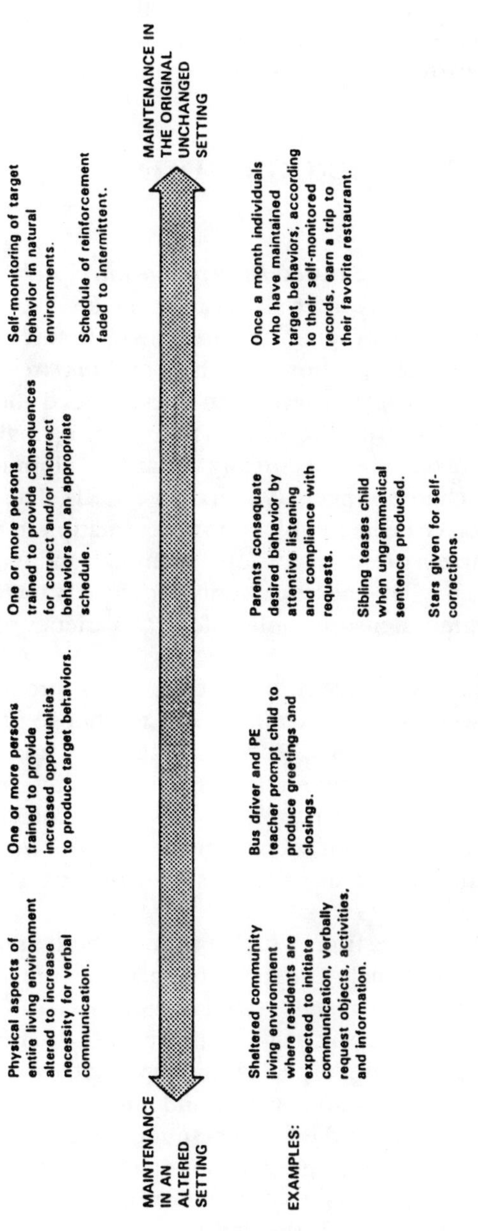

Figure 7–2. Continuum of varieties of maintenance, with examples.

Some issues pertinent to maintenance of language behaviors have been presented. Two kinds of maintenance, planned and unplanned, have been described, and the notion of natural maintaining contingencies has been discussed. In the next section, suggestions for achieving maintenance of learned behaviors will be presented.

SUGGESTIONS FOR PROGRAMMING MAINTENANCE

In their small booklet entitled *How to Maintain Behavior*, Kazdin and Esveldt-Dawson (1981) offer six basic procedures to maintain behavior after a treatment program is withdrawn. Before maintenance procedures are implemented, however, these authors stress that the behavior must be at an acceptable level, that is, established and stable. Two additional sources that offer suggestions for achieving maintenance of target behaviors are directed specifically toward developmentally disabled and autistic children (Egel, 1981; Lovaas, 1981). The suggestions by these authors have been combined for presentation in this section. Table 7–1 summarizes these suggestions. Although some of them may seem extreme and might be necessary only for severely involved clients, the principles behind them are applicable to all varieties of clients and behaviors.

An important initial suggestion to consider in programming for maintenance as well as for generalization is to choose functional behaviors as targets (Lovaas, 1981). Teach language, play, and self-help behaviors that result in important reinforcers within many environments. Choosing academic test information may result in achieving criterion on some standardized test, but such language behavior may serve little purpose in the child's everyday life. In such cases, we should expect little maintenance.

A rather global suggestion, which applies to both antecedent and consequent events, is to make the transition between the treatment environments "imperceptibly small" (Lovaas, 1981, p. 111). Create multiple environments in such a way that the child cannot discriminate when he or she is not in treatment. As part of this approach, parents and other persons frequently encountered by the child must become teachers, so that there is no vacation from therapy. These additional teachers manipulate both antecedent events (to provide opportunities for display of the target) and consequent events (to provide natural maintaining contingencies) when in contact with the child.

The training of such significant others is discussed further by Egel (1981). Three groups of individuals—peers, parents, and classroom

Table 7–1. Suggestions for Programming Maintenance

1. Choose functional language behaviors as targets, ones for which there exists a natural community of reinforcers that can serve as maintaining contingencies within nontreatment environments.
2. Make the transition between the treatment environment and other environments imperceptibly small. Make it difficult for clients to discriminate between treatment and nontreatment situations.
3. Teach peers, parents, and classroom teachers to provide antecedent events for display of the language target and to deliver appropriate consequent events for correct and incorrect production.
4. Avoid artificial or contrived reinforcers that are not likely to be found in nontreatment environments, such as candy, points, or tokens. Try to determine some naturally occurring contingencies for the target behavior and use them as the behavior becomes more stable.
5. Gradually change from immediate reinforcement to delayed reinforcement by introducing brief delays before delivering reinforcement.
6. Extend a low-powered version of the treatment program into new situations, perhaps by involving others to provide prompts and praise on an intermittent schedule. Gradually fade out the program as maintenance is noted.

teachers—may be included in plans for programming maintenance. Consider developing peer support for the language target behavior. Not only are peer attention and approval powerful natural reinforcers, but many times situations can be arranged whereby peers directly provide consequences to the target child. For example, if peers share the reinforcement of special privileges earned by the target child, those peers begin to support and encourage the desired behaviors. Since those peers are part of the child's natural environments, such support may continue after the direct treatment is discontinued.

A problem that must be dealt with in training these people to apply programmed maintenance is how to ensure maintenance of *their* teaching behaviors. Research has hardly begun to address this issue, although such encouragers as course credit for teachers and fast-food coupons for parents have been tried. It is quite easy to imagine, of course, that the trained teaching behaviors would remain as long as contingencies were applied to them but would not be maintained without them—a repetition of the maintenance problem with the child's behaviors!

A second group of suggestions centers on reinforcers or rewards. Avoidance of artificial reinforcers that are not found outside school or therapy environments, such as candy, points, or tokens, is important, especially during generalization and maintenance phases of the treatment program. Parents may use these artificial reinforcers initially, but they should "normalize" rewards as soon as possible (Lovaas, 1982, p. 112). Social stimuli, such as praise, smiles, and physical contact, have been suggested as more natural reinforcers to replace artificial or contrived rewards. Unfortunately, such stimuli may not serve as natural maintaining contingencies if they are not frequently found outside the treatment environment. It may be necessary to pair artificial and social reinforcers at first, then fade out the artificial reinforcer as the social one becomes a conditioned reinforcer. Then we must ensure that those social gestures and phrases do indeed occur in natural environments.

In addition to the choice of reinforcer, use of a thin and intermittent schedule of reinforcement is advised, especially if artificial reinforcers must be continued. Of course, the schedule should only be changed during generalization or maintenance phases, *after* the target behavior has been well established. One way of making treatment and nontreatment environments more similar is to gradually reduce the frequency of reinforcement to an intermittent schedule. This, of course, may be done while a more direct treatment program is in effect and is useful as a generalization strategy also. Such intermittent reinforcement schedules must also be taught to, and applied by, significant others involved in the maintenance program. For some behaviors, however, a very thin schedule of reinforcement in the nontreatment environment may not be appropriate. For example, requests for desired objects or activities may be granted on nearly a one-to-one schedule, if the requests are reasonable. Even when requests are denied, a verbal explanation for the denial may be given, and this may serve as a maintaining contingency also.

Delaying reinforcement, again a suggestion to promote generalization across other parameters, can also be used to increase the similarity between treatment and other environments. Gradually change from immediate reinforcement to delayed reinforcement by introducing brief delays before applying the reinforcer. Contingencies should be faded so that there is a less direct connection between target behaviors and immediate rewards.

One final procedure for achieving maintenance, advocated by Kazdin and Esveldt-Dawson (1981), is extending a low-powered version of treatment into new situations to maintain or generalize the target behaviors in those new situations. Although behaviors produced under these conditions should not technically be called "maintained," it may be that a short period of programmed maintenance will lead to true maintenance of the target behaviors in the absence of treatment.

Now that a number of suggestions for achieving planned and unplanned maintenance of language target behaviors have been reviewed, several studies of language treatment, which have included some kinds of maintenance measures, will be summarized. The reader should consider whether any of the measurement methods or treatment procedures could be useful for the clients on his or her caseload.

STUDIES THAT INCLUDED MAINTENANCE MEASURES

The practical limitations of extensive follow-up measures after a period of successful treatment have resulted in a gap in the language intervention literature. Most intervention studies have not included a follow-up or maintenance measure. Tables 7–2 and 7–3 summarize a number of studies of language treatment that included maintenance measures of some kind. Notice the variability in the time periods between treatment termination and maintenance measures. Note also the number of maintenance measures obtained. It is difficult to reach any firm conclusions about the nature of maintenance of language behaviors in language-disordered populations owing to the variability in research methods and the definitions of maintenance.

Maintenance in Institutionalized MR Adults

The first three studies summarized in Table 7–2 were carried out with institutionalized mentally retarded adults. Target behaviors were signed requests by profoundly retarded adults in the first study. Positive social language behaviors were increased and negative social language behaviors were decreased in the other two studies.

Signed requests for objects or activities were taught to four profoundly retarded adults in a study reported by Duker and Morsink (1984). Details of this study have been described in previous chapters. A single maintenance measure three months after training ended showed various levels of maintenance among the four subjects. Two of the subjects showed 100 per cent maintenance of the three or four signs trained, whereas the other two subjects had lost some of the trained signs.

Table 7–2. Studies of Language Treatment that Have Included Maintenance Measures

Authors	Subjects	Language Target	Results
Duker and Morsink (1984)	4 profoundly MR institutionalized adults	Signed requests for objects and activities, e.g., pegs for pegboard, listening to music	At 3 months, some signs were maintained in nontreatment settings; one subject maintained 2 of 4 signs, a second maintained 4 of 4; a third maintained 1 of 3; and a fourth maintained 3 of 3
Foxx, McMurrow, and Mannemeier (1984)	6 institutionalized MR adults	Six verbal social skills, e.g., compliments, politeness, criticism	Weekly videotapes in workshop setting continued for 1 month after treatment; considerable variability; generalization/maintenance failure concluded
Matson and Earnhart (1981)	4 institutionalized MR adults	Language behaviors agreed upon by two staff members, e.g., loud talking, making derogatory comments, perseverative statements	Decreases in undesired behaviors were maintained on checks at 1 and 4 months after treatment
Lovaas, Koegel, Simmons, and Stevens-Long (1973)	13 autistic children	Appropriate speech	On 1- to 4-year follow-up measures in institution and home, 9 showed maintenance or improvement, and 4 lost treatment gains
Carr and Kologinsky (1983)	6 autistic children	Spontaneous signed requests for foods and activities	During maintenance measures for 19 to 24 sessions, spontaneous signing was maintained at 70–85% for 2 of 3 subjects; for 3 different subjects, maintenance of generalized signing across new adults was inconsistent; need for new adults to reinforce sign requests was concluded
Handleman (1981)	6 autistic children	One-word answers to questions involving common objects and actions, e.g., "What do you sit on?" in sets of 5 questions	For up to 5 probes after treatment had ceased, 3 children maintained responses, 1 showed a slight decrease, and 2 maintained few responses
Koegel and Rincover (1977)	6 autistic children	Receptive language targets, e.g., to imitate gestures and touch body parts	Comparison of various reinforcement schedules revealed that the thinner the schedule in treatment, the greater the maintenance in extra-therapy settings, and that intermittent noncontingent reinforcement increased durability of treatment gains
Gaylord-Ross, Haring, Breen, and Pitts-Conway (1984)	3 autistic youths	Verbal social initiations and interactions with normal high school students	At 4 months, 2 of 3 subjects maintained social interaction skills

For the six higher-functioning adults studied by Foxx, McMorrow, and Mennemeier (1984), several verbal social skills were taught. Treatment procedures were effective in achieving generalization to workshop simulations. During treatment and for four weeks after treatment had ceased, weekly videotapes were recorded in the actual workshop setting, thus providing setting generalization and maintenance measures. Four of the six adults' appropriate interactions were highest during the follow-up videotapes, and there was considerable variability in their responding. In addition, some residents showed a downward trend during the treatment phase. Therefore, the investigators concluded that the behaviors measured during the four weeks after treatment could not be considered effects of the training program. Generalization (or maintenance) failure was concluded.

The maintenance measure used in another study of mentally retarded residents of an institution was an example of programmed maintenance. For this study, which is described in greater detail in Chapter 8, one of the treatment phases included on-ward training of pairs of residents, along with training using scenes, in a therapy room. When staff members observed a target behavior (e.g., loud talking, making derogatory comments) that was not self-recorded by the resident, that staff member would contact the trainer immediately. The trainer would then administer training procedures (e.g., performance feedback, modeling, social reinforcement, role playing) to the resident at the spot where the misbehavior occurred. For the maintenance phase, on-ward sessions were held one and four months after treatment.

Results of this study indicated that once target behaviors had been decelerated for several days, gains were maintained by prompting on the ward without the necessity of training sessions in the therapy room. Maintenance required only a small amount of staff time, since target behaviors remained at low frequencies compared to baseline (Matson and Earnhart, 1981). However, all four subjects showed a rising trend for at least one of the target behaviors. Whether or not behaviors would increase to their baseline levels, thus showing extinction of treatment effects, is unknown. The programmed maintenance observed in this study involved cooperation of ward staff, who would contact the trainer or provide praise for self-monitoring or self-reporting. Apparently, the trainer was usually available within the setting.

These three studies of mentally retarded adults included maintenance measures that differed widely in the ways they were collected. Given these differences and differences in the kinds of behaviors trained, it is difficult to conclude anything regarding the maintenance results. None of the studies showed perfect maintenance across all subjects, but perhaps this is not a reasonable expectation.

Maintenance in Autistic Children or Youths

Five of the studies shown in Table 7–2 were carried out with autistic children or youths as subjects. Three of them included treatment procedures that have been mentioned as strategies for achieving generalization and maintenance effects, such as parent training (Lovaas et al., 1973) and training in multiple settings (Carr and Kologinsky, 1983; Handleman, 1981). Others describe the effects of different reinforcement schedules (Koegel and Rincover, 1977) and the use of normal high school peers as part of training (Gaylord-Ross, Haring, Breen, and Pitts-Conway, 1984).

The results of the Lovaas and co-workers (1973) study were described earlier, in Chapters 4 and 5. After language and other complex behaviors were taught to several autistic children, a comprehensive loss of those behaviors was noted two years after termination of treatment for those children released into institutions. Re-teaching resulted in recovery of the earlier gains, but again, behaviors were not maintained when nontreatment environments did not support them. By contrast, children released to trained parents did maintain treatment gains.

The studies by Carr and Kologinsky (1983) and Handleman (1981) included a strategy of training in multiple settings to increase the chance of generalization or maintenance. The six autistic children in the Carr and Kologinsky study were taught to produce signs as labels in response to "What is it?" or "What am I doing?" questions in pretraining sessions, and thus establishment of signs was not the treatment goal. Rather, the goals were to achieve spontaneous (unprompted) signing to request reinforcers, to investigate the relationship between spontaneous signing and self-stimulatory behaviors, and to identify variables that could produce generalization across settings and adults.

In their first experiment, Carr and Kologinsky built in a maintenance component, a phase identical to the baseline phase except that spontaneous signed requests were consequated with the reinforcer specified by the sign. This can be viewed as a programmed maintenance strategy, an example of applying natural reinforcing (maintenance) contingencies, since requests are often granted in natural environments. During four of the maintenance sessions, two nontraining persons were present but did not prompt signed requests. Results indicated that maintenance of the signs was observed even after the training component was discontinued. Anecdotal reports of classroom teachers indicated that the children were signing to request foods and activities, some of which had not been explicitly taught.

In their second experiment, Carr and Kologinsky (1983) included baseline trials in five generalization settings: a cafeteria area, two auxiliary classrooms, the gymnasium, and a hallway near the gymnasium. Treatment phases consisted of prompting and reinforcement of the first sign only, then of the second sign only, followed by a repetition of these two phases. A final phase consisted of treatment of both signs. Assessment of generalization across both settings and persons (within the treatment setting) occurred during the final sessions of each phase. Thus, extra trials were carried out within a play area, the art room, the school entrance, the psychological testing room, and a workshop area. Although reinforcement for correct signing did not occur, these were considered training trials during the treatment phase. Initially, one of the three subjects showed discrimination between the trainer and several nontrainers who did not deliver the requested objects. In this case, the nontrainer began to reinforce signing.

Results of this second experiment clearly indicated that spontaneity of signed requests generalized to new settings for the three children treated. The authors concluded that for maintenance to occur, however, adults in the new settings must reinforce the signs by delivering the objects specified.

These two experiments taken together argue for application of several procedures to achieve spontaneous production of signed requests in new settings. Spontaneity of signing appears to require opportunities for child-initiated communication, a characteristic of the incidental teaching strategy. Although discrete-trial training procedures may be effective in teaching language forms, such as labels, a dispersed-trial strategy with emphasis on child-initiated communication is more effective in achieving spontaneous language use, such as requesting behaviors. The two strategies are seen as complementary rather than antagonistic methods for facilitating language learning.

In the achievement of generalization to multiple settings and persons, training in several settings and choosing common stimuli (adults who appeared in the generalization settings) appeared to be contributing factors. In addition, the choice of signs was functional for the children; that is, children wanted the objects and activities signed for.

A final point made by Carr and Kologinsky (1983) directly relates to maintenance and measures of maintenance. When nontrainer adults did not reinforce signs in the generalization settings, maintenance of generalization was inconsistent across children. Even those who showed some maintenance would probably have ceased their spontaneous signing as requests were not granted. Thus, as the experimental data indicated, "... the most reliable procedure for maintaining generalized responding across new adults is to have these adults reinforce sign requests" (Carr and Kologinsky, 1983, p. 311). Indeed, this seems to be what adults normally do in response to requests in natural environments, provided that requests are reasonable. Thus, such responses would constitute natural maintaining contingencies, even if they are applied on a rather thick schedule.

Like the second experiment by Carr and Kologinsky, a study by Handleman (1981) included training in multiple settings. However, the results were not so encouraging. The Handleman study was designed to investigate the effects of two types of treatment on generalization of answers to one-word questions from clinic to a day-care setting. Each set of five questions was repeatedly probed after treatment criterion was met, thus allowing a measure of maintenance as well as setting generalization. Whether treatment occurred within restricted or multiple settings in the clinic made no difference in generalization across person (day-care teacher) and setting or in response maintenance for the six autistic children treated. For three of the children, responses, although not all at 100 per cent accuracy, showed no evidence of extinction for up to five probes after treatment. One child continued to respond at high levels, but a slight decrement was noted. The remaining two children maintained few responses.

Unfortunately, the period over which posttreatment probes continued was not given in this study (Handleman, 1981), but it was probably rather short. This was not a rigorous measure of maintenance. However, Handleman concluded that for some children, generalization of verbal responses across instructional settings may be somewhat resistant to extinction, that is, may be maintained. The results of this study did not support a strategy of training in multiple settings to facilitate generalization or maintenance, however.

The effects of various reinforcement schedules on maintenance of learned receptive language behaviors in six autistic children were investigated by Koegel and Rincover (1977). The results of this study provide support for suggestions to use thin schedules of reinforcement as a strategy for maintenance. After behaviors were acquired, each child was given additional (extra-therapy) trials on one of three reinforcement schedules: continuous reinforcement, fixed ratio of two-to-one, or fixed ratio of five-to-one. To assess durability of responding, trials were conducted by a stranger in the extra-therapy setting until correct responding either decreased to 0 per cent or was maintained at 80 per cent for at least 100 consecutive trials. In addition to the three schedules previously described, effects of noncontingent reinforcement in the extra-therapy environment were also assessed for two children whose responding had extinguished (decreased to 0 per cent) and for two additional children. The noncontingent reinforcement was administered 10 seconds after either ten incorrect responses or 20 trials, as the stranger gave the child a piece of candy. Additional trials were then presented.

Results indicated that the thinner the reinforcement schedule, the greater the maintenance of treatment gains in extra-therapy settings; e.g., a child on the five-to-one schedule continued responding at 80 per cent accuracy for as many as 500 trials. Results for the noncontingent reinforcement indicated that intermittent use of noncontingent reinforcers in the extra-therapy setting further increased the durability of treatment gains. For example, two children receiving noncontingent rewards after every 20 trials continued to respond for 440 to 540 trials before the behavior extinguished. Given that the behaviors taught were not particularly functional and that reinforcers were artificial, these results are impressive. Certainly schedules of reinforcement are an important consideration in programming maintenance. Whether similar results would be observed for more functional target behaviors and when reinforcers were less artificial is not known.

The final study described in this section sought to increase social initiations and the duration of social interactions of two autistic and retarded youths (Gaylord-Ross, Haring, Breen, and Pitts-Conway, 1984). Training occurred in both a special education classroom and in an outdoor courtyard that was also used to assess person generalization, at times when normal high school students took a break there. The following five experimental conditions were used to assess effects of training: (1) an initial baseline condition, (2) an object-only condition where subjects only carried desirable objects (e.g., hand-held video game, Sony Walkman radio, gum), (3) object function training, (4) social-skill training, which included language behaviors, and (5) maintenance at four months posttreatment. During the social-skill training condition, six peer trainers were rotated across sessions; these students were not among those present for generalization probes.

The training in object function and in verbal social skills—i.e., greetings, offering to play with the object with the peer, and a termination response—was successful in achieving acquisition and generalization of social initiations and interactions across peers not involved in treatment. For example, subjects were initiating interactions with normal peers at a rate of one to three encounters in a 15-minute break period. The maintenance measure, taken after summer vacation, showed that two of the subjects maintained skills, although with lower frequency. Gaylord-Ross and associates speculated that maintenance failure by the third subject may have been due to forgetting the skills over the summer or to the fact that familiar peers from the past school year were not present in the fall.

In discussing their results, Gaylord-Ross and co-workers (1984) pointed out the importance of identifying the kinds of settings and persons to which trained behaviors should generalize. Although some social verbal initiations may be appropriate with unfamiliar persons, more often individuals communicate with familiar persons in familiar settings. Clinicians should ask themselves where and with whom the target language behaviors they have chosen should be maintained. In some cases, the behaviors may be appropriate to specific settings and persons, but not to all. In these instances, clients may need to be taught to discriminate between appropriate and inappropriate situations to produce the target language behavior.

The use of interesting and desirable objects, which might provoke comment and conversation from peers, was a strategy used by Gaylord-Ross and colleagues that could prove useful with many language-deficient clients. These objects could be viewed as topics for conversation and perhaps as mediators of conversational language behavior, if they serve as common antecedents for language within various non-treatment environments. Certainly, the study by Gaylord-Ross and associates suggests several ideas for generalization and maintenance of social language behaviors that are worth pursuing.

Maintenance in Language-Disordered Children

The three studies described in this section include targets such as grammatical features or rules and frequency of verbalizations, which were chosen for young language-delayed children. Time periods for maintenance measures ranged from three-and-a-half weeks to four months. Table 7–3 summarizes these studies of young language-disordered children that included maintenance measures.

In the Culatta and Horn (1982) study, the goal was generalization of grammar targets that had achieved 100 per cent accuracy criterion on structured probes to spontaneous discourse. Maintenance measures were collected within treatment sessions. Within the multiple-baseline design across two grammar targets per child, a four-step program (described in more detail in Chapter 4) was applied until criterion was met, i.e., 90 per cent correct production in the first ten obligatory contexts for two consecutive sessions. Individual therapy sessions of 45 minutes occurred twice weekly.

Maintenance measures for initially trained targets were computed after treatment procedures for that target were terminated. These targets showed maintenance at 90 per cent accuracy on measures obtained at least seven sessions after treatment had ceased. Although this was only about three-and-a-half weeks, it is an encouraging indication that maintenance of grammar targets within spontaneous discourse does occur. The four-step program employed five evoking strategies designed

Table 7–3. Studies of Language-deficient Children that Included Maintenance Measures

Authors	Subjects	Language Target	Results
Culatta and Horn (1982)	4 language-disordered children	Grammar targets, e.g., *is, am, will, went,* and *not,* in conversational speech	Probes within treatment sessions 7 sessions after training on the target had ceased showed maintenance at 90% accuracy in spontaneous discourse
Rogers-Warren and Warren (1980)	3 language-deficient children	Rate of verbalization, novel word combinations, and grammar targets learned in therapy	At 4 months, follow-up measures for 3 months showed that 2 of 3 subjects maintained targets on classroom measures; no data available for third subject
Warren, McQuarter, and Rogers-Warren (1984)	3 language-delayed children	Obligatory and nonobligatory verbalizations	For up to 2 months, rates of verbalization were maintained at above-baseline rates after teachers had reduced frequency of mands and models to prompt child speech
Campbell & Stremel-Campbell (1982)	2 moderately language-delayed children	*Is* and *are* in *wh-* questions, yes-no questions, and statements learned during academic tasks	A maintenance program of social reinforcement for spontaneous target production and a VR3 token schedule was applied to initial targets while training continued on subsequent targets; data suggested that these contingencies were adequate to maintain correct production

to provide opportunities for using the grammar targets. No specific consequences for correct productions were described, but errors in production were consequated by the clinician's responding to the intent of the message and expanding the incorrect rule form. The role that contingencies played in achievement of maintenance is unclear. Apparently, provision of antecedent events was the primary teaching strategy, and some kind of natural maintaining contingencies were operating to reinforce correct production during maintenance measures.

The two additional studies described in this section employed similar teaching approaches (Rogers-Warren and Warren, 1980; Warren, McQuarter, and Rogers-Warren, 1984). The mand-model procedure, a modified version of Hart and Risley's incidental teaching procedure, allows the teacher to initiate an episode for teaching as well as child-initiated episodes for incidental teaching.

Language targets for the study by Rogers-Warren and Warren (1980) included rates of verbalization, novel word combinations, and grammatical features. Details of this procedure were described in Chapters 5 and 6. Application of this procedure clearly accelerated the display of language targets learned in one-to-one training and resulted in increases in the overall rate and complexity of language in the classroom. In addition, long-term follow-up measures available for two subjects showed that verbalization rates remained high for three monthly probes implemented four months after treatment. The authors suggested that the children's increased frequency of talking brought them into contact with natural reinforcers, possibly adult attention, available for language use. These natural reinforcers found in the classroom then served to maintain verbalization rates.

In addition to measuring child verbalization rates, the second study (Warren, McQuarter, and Rogers-Warren, 1984) measured teacher rates of mands and models. From very low verbalization rates during baseline, rates for all three children increased substantially during mand-model intervention to levels approximateing those observed in normal peers. During the maintenance condition, when rates of instructions to verbalize (mands) and models decreased, all three children maintained or increased their rates of verbalization. The authors noted that use of the mand-model procedure may have sensitized the teachers to specific needs of the children, increasing overall teacher-child interaction rates. Perhaps the increase in appropriate child responses served to reinforce the *teacher's* verbal behavior, a possible natural maintaining contingency for teacher interactions.

An interesting unanticipated effect of the Warren and associates study was that the three children's MLUs continued to increase during the maintenance condition, which followed an intervention phase in which two-word rather than single-word responses were required. Apparently, longer utterances increased in frequency, even after teacher mands and models were decreased. This might indicate that whatever natural maintaining contingencies were operating during the maintenance condition might have differentially affected *longer* utterances.

These two studies of the effects of a mand-model version of incidental teaching support the value of this approach as a strategy for generalization and maintenance of language behaviors. As was discussed in Chapter 3, incidental teaching can have a domino effect, with an initial increase in just the frequency of talking resulting in more elaborated and complex language as rates of verbalization increase.

One final study that included a maintenance measure was also described in Chapter 5. A "loose training" strategy was used to teach production of grammar targets during academic tasks to two moderately delayed children. A programmed maintenance strategy was instituted for each target after it was acquired, while the next target was trained. The maintenance program consisted of social reinforcement for spontaneously produced correct productions and three-to-one variable schedule of token reinforcement. Unlike the earlier treatment phase, prompts were not used during the maintenance condition. Thus, during the maintenance program, only consequent events were manipulated.

Results indicated that for the first subject, frequency of correct productions of the first target (*is* and *are* in *wh-* questions) declined during maintenance phase but remained considerably higher than frequency of incorrect productions, which also declined after formal training had ended. The data suggested that placing contingencies on the first target was adequate to maintain correct use while a second target was trained. Data for the second subject also showed that frequency of correct responses remained consistently higher than errors. Thus, the maintenance program of intermittent reinforcement for correct responses appeared to be successful in keeping errors low in frequency, but not in keeping correct productions high in frequency.

Since grammatically correct *is* and *are* should eventually reach a criterion of 90 to 100 per cent in obligatory contexts to be considered normal, it would have been quite interesting to continue maintenance measures as contingencies were faded to see if errors would eventually approach zero frequencies. Since even during the treatment phase of this study, error rates did not reach zero frequency, it seems unlikely that 100 per cent grammatical production would have occurred.

The study included a programmed maintenance strategy and a loose training strategy, both of which should facilitate generalization and maintenance. However, the continued use of token reinforcement, even on a variable schedule, runs counter to suggestions made earlier in this chapter concerning the avoidance of artificial reinforcers.

The four studies of maintenance of language target behaviors in language-deficient children suggested that achievement of maintenance is possible. None of the studies, however, employed what could be considered a rigorous measure of maintainence, i.e., unobtrusive observation of the client in a variety of nontreatment situations. Compared with the results of maintenance in studies of other language-deficient populations, however, results of these studies are encouraging.

SUMMARY

The long-term maintenance of language behaviors learned in treatment is an important goals of clinical intervention. Behaviors that have generalized appropriately, i.e., to the right settings and persons, must be maintained in nontreatment environments, or the time and effort spent in teaching them will have been wasted.

Among the suggestions for maintenance presented in this chapter were several that should be considered from the very beginning of treatment and some that should be considered as the language targets begin to show some generalization across various parameters. By choosing functional target behaviors, the clinician can improve the chances for maintenance, since useful behaviors are often those that receive reinforcement in many nontreatment settings. Any ways that the conditions of treatment and nontreatment can be made more similar will increase chances for both generalization and maintenance. By involving peers, parents, and classroom teachers in the provision of antecedent events that set the occasion for display of the language target, and by teaching these significant others to deliver appropriate, natural reinforcing contingencies for the target, many nontreatment situations can take on treatment aspects.

Finally, special attention must be paid to the kinds of reinforcement used during the final stages of treatment, as well as to the schedules of reinforcement used. Remember that some kind of natural maintaining contingencies must be operating for any behavior to continue. Those natural contingencies should be tapped as part of a programmed maintenance strategy.

Now that a number of maintenance strategies have been presented and discussed, the reader may have discovered some viable, workable ideas to try with clients. In the final chapter, some specific ideas for implementing generalization and maintenance strategies will be offered, with special attention to the role of parents and the possibility of self-monitoring and mediation strategies.

Chapter 8

Implementing Generalization Strategies

The reader may have been considering the information presented in the various studies discussed in the previous chapters in light of present clients and their generalization patterns. Some of the procedures that have worked in achieving generalization in these studies may seem worth a try. The purpose of this last chapter is to pull out some of the most effective procedures described as facilitators of generalization and to present them in ways that allow them to be incorporated into the clinician's therapy plans.

It may be apparent by now that including generalization strategies at the end of the establishment phase of therapy may not be the best way to go. If this book has had its intended impact, clinicians will reformulate their approaches to language intervention and place the goal of appropriate generalization very early in the game plan. From the first day of treatment, some of the generalization strategies can be started.

DIFFERENCES BETWEEN ESTABLISHMENT AND GENERALIZATION STRATEGIES

Because of the differences between initial learning and later generalization of target behaviors, there are differences in procedures used to *establish* a behavior and those used to facilitate *generalization* of that behavior. Herein lies the "clinician's dilemma." Some of the conditions of treatment required for initial acquisition of a behavior are not conducive to generalization of that behavior.

The purpose of an establishment phase of treatment is to get a particular behavioral unit—i.e., the language target—into the client's repertoire, that is, to ensure that the client can produce it in response to certain stimuli. In order to do that, treatment conditions have to be more controlled than generalization conditions. For example, during the establishment phase the format of therapy may have to be highly structured; frequent repetitions may be required; stimulus materials and antecedent events may need to be unvaried from trial to trial; and frequent and consistent application of consequent events for correct and incorrect productions may be necessary. These features of treatment might be called *establishment procedures*, and they should work quite efficiently in establishing a high rate of accurate productions of the target—a strong response. However, if treatment does not result automatically in a generalized response, then these establishment features of treatment must be changed. They are by and large *not* conducive to achieving generalization.

It may be that, for some clients, the initial learning conditions need not be so highly structured. Preschool classrooms in which antecedent and consequent events do not appear to be rigidly structured may be conducive to a great deal of learning and generalization for some children. Part of the problem is deciding how to measure learning of target behaviors and generalization of that learning. If specific targets are measured by structured probes, little learning may be revealed after intervention that is not highly structured. However, if more global measures of language learning are made—for instance, performance on various language tests or inventories—then loosely structured environments may result in much improvement. Perhaps language learning will take longer under less structured conditions, but the behaviors that are learned will generalize better. Controlled research needs to be done to investigate such possibilities.

At present we may only speculate that individual clients may learn better under differing degrees of structure and that the kinds of language targets chosen may influence the degree of structure used to teach them. When it is necessary to control the treatment format tightly to achieve the desired behavior change, it is important that the structure be loosened as soon as it is feasible. Otherwise, the desired behavior may be produced only in the artificial, highly structured treatment environment and may never transfer to the loosely structured natural environment.

APPLYING GENERALIZATION PRINCIPLES

Early in Chapter 1 a list of Stokes and Baer's (1977) generalization tactics was presented. Since that 1977 review, a number of other authors have addressed the generalization problem, enlarging on and interpreting some of the tactics presented by Stokes and Baer. The brief review of suggestions for facilitating generalization that follows is a synthesis of ideas from a number of sources (Baer, 1981; Carr, 1980; Kazdin, 1978;

Spradlin and Siegel, 1982; Stokes and Baer, 1977). Some of these suggestions involve decisions that should be made right at the beginning of intervention, such as the choice of functional language targets. Others should be considered later, after some progress has been made during an establishment phase of treatment. Consider how the following principles might be applied to clients who exhibit problems in generalization of language target behaviors.

1. **Choose functional targets.** As language targets, select behaviors that will be useful (i.e., functional) for the client in many natural environments. These will have a high probability of generalizing because they will meet a natural community of reinforcement.
2. **Teach enough examples.** Do not expect generalization after teaching only one example to criterion. The necessary range of examples may vary from 10 to 200, depending on the individual and the behavior.
3. **Choose the *best* examples to teach.** Think about the components of the generalized behavior that is the goal and pick examples that include those components.
4. **Teach a few examples simultaneously.** Try one or two trials with one example, then one or two with another example. Avoid massed trial training with only one example.
5. **Teach loosely.** Loosen the control over stimuli in the teaching sessions and the consequent events following opportunities to respond. Decrease the structure of the teaching situations to make them more similar to natural environments.
6. **Vary the antecedents.** Do not allow any *one* stimulus to gain control over the target behavior. Use important, transportable stimuli (e.g., parents, peers) that are common to both the teaching situation and the generalization situations.
7. **Vary the consequences**. Make the reinforcement schedule and the reinforcers similar to the variety of consequences that occur in the natural environment. Work toward a thin, intermittent schedule of reinforcement, or delay it to increase the chance that the behavior will be maintained after treatment has ceased.
8. **Program the natural environment.** Restructure some aspects of the natural environment in such a way as to support the target behavior. This can involve increasing the opportunities for the behavior to occur as well as increasing the probability that the behavior will be effective (reinforced) when it does occur.
9. **Teach self-monitoring.** Use self-monitoring and verbal mediation where possible so that the client becomes both a stimulus for and a reinforcer of the target behavior. Teach clients to observe and report accurately their performance on the language targets.

A number of these principles, while suggested by experience, lack experimental validation. As more research is focused on investigating factors that influence generalization subsequent to treatment, these principles may become more clearly defined.

In thinking about applying these nine strategies, it may be useful to designate when, in the course of intervention, each may be considered. The first one, choosing functional targets, must be considered at the very beginning of treatment. The second, third, and fourth strategies should be considered during the establishment phase of treatment, and the remaining strategies can be considered as the focus of treatment shifts toward achievement of generalization. As generalization checks reveal that targets are not generalizing as desired, treatment strategies must focus on making the treatment and natural environments more similar.

There are basically two options for increasing the similarity between these two environments and thus achieving generalization. The speech-language clinician can make either the therapy setting more like the natural environment or the natural environment more like the therapy setting. Of course, a combination of both may be more feasible as well as more effective.

Let us take the first option, making the therapy setting similar to the natural environment, and illustrate how the language therapy that takes place in a confined, artificial, often highly structured setting can be altered so that it simulates some aspects of the natural environments where generalization of language behaviors is desired. Table 8–1 lists five ways in which various aspects of therapy may be changed so that therapy becomes more similar to natural environments. First, the physical attributes of the setting can be altered. Second, the visual stimulus materials used to elicit language responses may be altered. Third, the language used by the clinician can be altered. Fourth, group interaction can be practiced. And fifth, the consequences that follow both correct and incorrect language produced by the client can be altered.

To implement the second option, making the natural environment more like the therapy setting, plans must be made to alter physical and social characteristics of one or more living, working, or playing environment. Table 8–2 lists five ways that various natural environments may be changed to incorporate some treatment characteristics. We may try to involve significant other people who frequently interact with the client in several natural environments. Parents and siblings may come to mind, as well as peers at school. Perhaps the verbal and nonverbal behaviors of these people can be altered in ways that will provide more opportunities to use the language target or in ways that will reinforce specific language behaviors with natural consequences. Perhaps some

Table 8–1. Ways to Make Therapy Situations More Like Natural Environments

1. Alter the physical attributes of the setting; e.g., move tables and chairs, add carpeting and posters, to simulate natural environments where the target language behaviors are expected to occur. Conduct therapy in a variety of nontherapy settings, e.g., hallways, classrooms, playground.
2. Alter the visual stimulus materials used; e.g., use photographs taken of the client in various places. Use popular magazines, toys, entertainment items (radio, stereo, watch, video game), board games, clothing, jewelry, grooming items.
3. Alter the language used by the clinician; e.g., reduce the frequency of direct instructions. Try role-playing various scenes that simulate experiences within a variety of natural environments.
4. Move from one-to-one interaction between clinician and client to small-group interaction. Use turn-taking in dialogues on a given topic, with feedback given to individuals after the dialogue is done or after a certain time period.
5. Use less direct and less artificial consequences for correct and incorrect production of the language target behaviors. Instead of verbal consequences such as "No, say 'She is baking a cake' " try a more subtle cue to prompt a self-correction of grammatical structure, such as "What did you say?" with a puzzled facial expression.

physical features of the environments can be changed, for example, making the living arrangements conducive to social language use or providing books, games, and even tape recorders that foster or require language use. These changes provide new visual stimuli that may serve as topics for talk and thus set the occasion for production of the language target. Finally, teaching a self-monitoring strategy to the client constitutes a change in natural environments, since the client takes that behavior outside of treatment. A careful observation and inventory of characteristics of the natural environments of the client can help clinicians decide how best to balance the two options—changing characteristics of the therapy situation and changing characteristics of natural environments.

In the following sections the major principles underlying specific suggestions for fostering generalization of language targets will be examined. Whether they will be implemented within treatment situations

Table 8–2. Ways to Make Natural Environments More Like Therapy Situations

1. Alter the verbal and nonverbal behaviors of parents, siblings, and other family members. For example, teach parents to ask the kinds of questions that will provide opportunities for display of the language target behavior. Teach parents and siblings to recognize and give positive responses to the language target and to ignore or give negative responses to errors in language target production.
2. Alter the verbal and nonverbal behaviors of peers, friends, teachers, and other people found frequently in nontreatment environments. For example, teach peers and teachers to provide prompts for production of language targets and to respond appropriately to correct and incorrect productions of language targets.
3. Alter the physical environment within the living space of the client. For example, the dining arrangements in group homes or the recreational spaces within institutional settings might be altered to provide more opportunities for display of the language target behaviors. Arrange the physical setting to promote social interaction among groups of clients or among clients and staff.
4. Alter the visual stimuli available to talk about. For example, plan to change toys or games available for recreation or plan and take trips to interesting places to provide topics for discussion and social interaction. Remember, we often talk about *new* information and events or *changes* in routines.
5. Teach the client self-monitoring and self-reinforcement behaviors that can be used within natural environments. This may include self-reminders to produce the language target — e.g., wearing a Band-Aid or marking a spot that will be noticed frequently — in order to remind the client to produce and monitor the behavior.

or outside of treatment in natural environments may be determined by individual clinicians and the clients involved. Some research not presented in earlier chapters will be reviewed and summarized as it relates to the generalization principles discussed.

Choosing Functional Targets

Functional responses can be defined as behaviors that occur naturally during a client's interaction with the environment and that produce an immediate consequence that is potentially reinforcing and specific (Guess, Sailor, and Baer, 1978). For example, requests are a class of language behaviors that, if generalized, should be quite useful in a variety of natural environments and often may result in the granting of the request. For a nonverbal or low-verbal child who gestures or has tantrums, a simple word (help) or sign to request assistance may be taught. Such a word or sign would be more easily interpreted by listeners, especially those who may not be very familiar with the child. For acquiring a desired object, two-word combinations may be required (*want/give + cookie*). Requests for information will require more sophisticated language structures, but these can be taught as the child acquires the necessary linguistic prerequisites and indicates cognitive readiness.

As children acquire a way to communicate messages such as "I can't do this" or "This task is too difficult," a reduction in aggressive and tantrum behavior may result (Carr, 1980). For example, a child who routinely displayed aggressive behavior when he had finished dinner and wished to leave the dining hall was taught a simple manual sign for "Let me out." When this alternative means of escaping from a place was learned, aggressive behavior decreased even though no contingencies were applied to it (Carr, Newsom, and Binkoff, 1980).

In attempting to apply this principle to choosing language targets for individual children, the clinician may want both to observe the child in several natural environments (classrooms, home) and to talk to significant others who frequently interact with the child. Observation can lead to an awareness of the kinds of language targets that would help the child to function more effectively in the various environments. Talking to parents can provide valuable input about the language targets that would be most appreciated (and therefore reinforced) by parents in nonschool environments.

As another example of choosing functional targets, consider a child who plays alone, does not interact socially with other children, and does not initiate language with adults but only responds when asked. To get a desired toy away from another child during free play, this child grabs it and conflict ensues. Perhaps a few socially appropriate requests would be a good target. "Can I play?" might be an appropriate choice if the child's language structure is sufficiently developed. Alternatively, a simpler phrase such as "truck, please" and offering another toy in exchange might be an appropriate choice for another child.

Choosing Examples to Teach

The second, third, and fourth principles listed earlier all address the choices of examples to teach. For language targets, classes of behavior are usually taught because we want a rule that applies to all members of that class to be learned. Even when we are teaching single words, we need to choose words that are not only functional, but that will readily combine with other words to generate two- and then three-word utterances. When considering examples to teach from a class of language target behaviors, we need to choose the best examples from the class and to teach several examples simultaneously. This holds true whether the target class is two- and three-word combinations, sentences, semantic classes, language functions, or conversational skills. After several examples are taught to some criterion level, probing for response generalization to untrained members of the class should be done, as well as probing for generalization to spontaneous production in natural environments.

Teaching Loosely

Loosening the structure of language therapy involves decreasing the control over antecedent and consequent events, thus leaving them more freedom to vary. Experimental studies of language intervention often maximize control over various factors that can affect language learning, such as number of trials, antecedent events, consequent events, reinforcement schedules, and possible distracting stimuli. By controlling such factors, researchers can discover the effects of changing one factor by holding all others constant. As discussed earlier, this results in a highly structured teaching method, which may be quite effective for *establishing* a target behavior, but not for generalizing it.

In clinical language teaching, tight control over many variables may be necessary initially to get the behavior into the child's repertoire. However, as soon as the child displays some control over the language target, the clinician's control over numerous variables must be reduced by varying antecedent and consequent events. Think about the characteristics of natural environments. Many different antecedents, in various combinations, will trigger language. Some will be verbal and some nonverbal. Consider the variety of consequent events that can follow language behavior. Sometimes we get the things we ask for; sometimes we don't. Sometimes a listener acknowledges our comments; sometimes our comments are ignored. Although conversation *is* structured, in the sense that certain conversational rules are followed, the structure does not resemble the structured teaching dialogues that characterize language therapy sessions. Since the natural environments to which the language target must generalize are often quite loosely structured, the degree of structure or control in language therapy must be reduced to resemble that of the natural environments if generalization is to occur.

Loosening the structure of language teaching sessions can be accomplished in numerous ways. Baer (1981) suggests using two or more teachers in two or more places, varying body positions, hand gestures, tone of voice, word choices, dress, lighting and noise levels, and even temperature and smells. Teaching several examples at once, rather than training to criterion on only one example, may also be considered a loosening of structure in language teaching. If the language target is produced accurately and consistently in therapy but does not occur or occurs at a low level outside the treatment environment, then something needs to be changed. Consider loosening the teaching technique in several ways.

Connell (1982), in presenting a strategy for helping language-disordered children figure out the rules for target grammatical structures, included the advice to train loosely in presenting stimulus pictures or objects to children to elicit target responses. Children should be exposed to changes in the stimuli as often as possible, in order to recognize the need to generalize beyond the materials used. However, his "contrast training" approach employed the same verbal antecedents (*wh-* questions) throughout all eight program steps. In the application of the "train loosely" principle, perhaps both verbal and visual stimuli should be changed frequently once the initial establishment phase is completed.

PROGRAMMING THE NATURAL ENVIRONMENT

Several aspects of the natural environment may be changed to facilitate generalization and maintenance of learned behaviors. Careful observation of the conditions that support desired language behaviors and those that undermine them is necessary before a decision is made on characteristics to alter. Three groups of people may come to mind as part of the environment that may be amenable to change. Parents of language-handicapped children are obvious targets, classroom peers are a second group to use in restructuring natural environments, and institutional staff may constitute an available group of people to recruit for clients in residential facilities.

Although other aspects of natural environments may also be amenable to change (e.g., physical barriers to communication, access to augmentative communication aids, planned social activities), it is the people available to communicate with who can provide major support within natural environments. The following sections provide examples of methods that have been used to restructure natural environments, using people available.

Parents as Language Teachers

Involving parents in the language treatment programs for their children is a way of applying two major principles of generalization. If parents are present during language teaching and are taught to provide stimuli (verbal or nonverbal) for eliciting the target language, then they are part of a "common stimulus." Since a parent is likely to be present during many of the child's experiences in natural environments, that presence may trigger appropriate language behaviors. Thus, parents can play a role in arranging for antecedent events to occur, which can increase the opportunities for producing language target behaviors.

Parents can also play a role in providing consequent events. When parents are taught to respond in specific ways to the presence or absence of language target behaviors, they become part of a natural community of reinforcement—a frequent source of feedback for both correct and incorrect language. For example, a parent may respond with a direct comment on the correct production of a target grammatical form at an early point in the generalization phase. At a later time, a parent may respond to a grammatical error with a more subtle "What did you say?" or a repetition of the error (e.g., "What that boy doing?") as a hint or prompt to self-correct. Thus, parents can contribute to generalization of language behaviors by being or providing common stimuli for language and by applying appropriate consequences for the desired language behaviors.

A number of behavior modification studies have involved parents in the teaching of language skills to their language-handicapped children (Arnold, Sturgis, and Forehand, 1977; Lovaas, Koegel, Simmons, and Long, 1973; Miller and Sloane, 1976; Muir and Milan, 1982; Wedel and Fowler, 1984). Parents can be effective forces in facilitating transfer of children's verbal skills to important natural environments and in ensuring reinforcement of those skills to maintain them. It is important to remember that transfer of behaviors can occur from home to school, as well as from school to home. Kyne (1980), in discussing the parent-professional relationship, provided an example of teachers establishing as an objective a behavior the child already showed as home. Rather than teach that behavior as though it were not in the child's repertoire, the teachers could approach it as a problem in generalization, applying strategies used by the parent at home. Frequent communication between parents and clinicians can increase the chances of succeeding as a team.

As many clinicians know from experience, however, not *all* parents may be willing or able to spend time learning to teach or transfer language targets. Thus, some care and good judgment must be exercised in deciding whether and when to involve parents in language treatment programs. Furthermore, parents do not want their children's programs to be contingent upon *their* ability or willingness to cooperate in a parent training program (Kyne, 1980).

If parents are to be involved in language teaching, the parents themselves must be taught. In addition, those parents' teaching skills should generalize across settings and time. The clinician's ultimate goal should be to change the parents' language and nonlanguage behaviors in such a way as to facilitate language development. If parents approach the task thinking that they are going to teach a specific language behavior to their child by method X during two 20-minute periods a week, it is unlikely that such teaching behavior will generalize. Instead, some general principles of language teaching must become part of the parents' behavioral repertoire, so that generalized language-teaching skills are available for use with the child throughout the day. Thus, some assessment of language interaction between parent and child must be done to determine general goals for parent language-teaching behavior.

The initial assessment of parent-child language interaction should include measures of language use and communication between the parent and the child. As part of a comprehensive language intervention program for preschoolers, Ruder, Bunce, and Ruder (1984) developed a rating sheet for parents to use as they learned language teaching skills. It includes specific behaviors to rate, such as getting the child's attention before talking, talking about the here and now, labeling objects and talking about actions, pausing to give the child opportunities to talk, responding meaningfully, expanding the child's utterances, and asking appropriate questions. After parents used the rating sheet to score teacher-child interaction on videotapes, parent-child videotapes were made and scored. Parents were then encouraged to use the sheet at home and were assigned specific activities such as direct training of a target language structure or recording data in the home.

For autistic children, an intensive parent training effort may be necessary. The effects of such intensive parent training were investigated by Koegel, Schreibman, Bitten, Burke, and O'Neill (1981). Two groups of 2- to 5-year-old autistic children were randomly assigned to two groups. For one group, child behaviors were treated by trained clinicians with no parent training provided; for the other group, child behaviors were treated by trained parents, with no clinic treatment provided. Parent training in behavior modification procedures was quite rigorous, including reading, observing videotape models of correct and incorrect use of procedures, practicing with feedback, and finally, taking a 15-minute structured criterion test that was scored in five skill areas. Details of the parent training procedures, which required an average of 5 to 10 weeks of five sessions per week, are described in Koegel and associates (1981).

To determine the effects of the two treatments on child behaviors, both generalization and maintenance measures were collected. A number of appropriate and inappropriate behaviors were noted both in structured laboratory observations with mother, therapist, and stranger and in home observations. Child behaviors included appropriate play and speech, social nonverbal behavior, tantrums, psychotic speech, self-stimulation, and noncooperation; thus, not all the target behaviors related to language. On a follow-up measure three months after treatment, the parent-trained children showed greater progress than the clinic-trained children, but not in the presence of a stranger. The parent-trained children also showed greater improvement on home observation measures. For both measures, the major difference between groups occurred between posttreatment and follow-up. Apparently, the parent training was particularly effective for maintenance. The investigators concluded that as much initial improvement, and more durable improvement, was observed with 25 to 50 hours of parent training as with 225 hours of direct clinic treatment. Certainly, parent training could be considered quite cost effective.

Some studies of parent teaching have looked for changes in the parent's language behaviors as well as changes in the child's language. Measures of generalization for parent language behavior should be built into research designed to investigate the effects of parent training on children's language learning. Suppose a parent teaching program has resulted in a child's successful learning of specific conversational skills as measured during treatment. If those child language behaviors do not generalize or are not maintained after treatment, it may be because the parent teaching behaviors that initially brought about those conversational skills did not generalize or were not maintained after treatment was terminated.

Studies that have investigated the effects of parent training are quite varied in their approaches and in the kinds of language behaviors targeted. In some studies, a parent was brought into the therapy room; in others, parents were trained at home; and sometimes both approaches were used.

In a study designed to modify antecedents and consequences applied by parents to the speech of their 6- to 12-year-old nonverbal children, Miller and Sloane (1976) trained five mother-child pairs in two home settings: a snack setting and a formal speech setting. The pairs were trained using a multiple-baseline design across pairs. During training, a wrist counter was given to the parent to record the number of times she prompted vocalizations during the snack. Feedback regarding parent behavior was also given immediately following the snack session. Parent training was terminated (i.e., no wrist counter or feedback) after the parent had increased her frequency of prompting and attending to speech by 50 per cent over baseline levels and could identify correct versus incorrect responses 80 per cent of the time in the formal speech setting. Generalization of parent and child behaviors was measured in a pre-snack setting at home and in a speech session and a free-play session at school.

Results indicated that parent prompting and attending immediately increased with training in the training settings. Parent prompting also generalized somewhat to the pre-snack setting; however, parent attending to vocalizations did not. Four of the five children showed small increases in vocalizations in the pre-snack setting. Generalization effects were not observed to the formal speech session at school, except for one child. Some increase in vocalizations during free play at school was noted, but it was not large. Miller and Sloane concluded that generalization of parent behaviors occurred only minimally, perhaps owing to incompatibilities between mothers' activities in the pre-snack setting and attending to their children's vocalizations. The authors questioned the usefulness of training parents under only one stimulus condition and suggested that generalization must be programmed.

For this study, it would have been interesting to find out what would have happened had the parents been allowed to keep the wrist counters. The counters may have functioned as mediators of the parent training language. Perhaps the mothers would have been reminded to produce the attending and praise behaviors as well as the prompts for speech. As for setting generalization, it was perhaps unreasonable to expect the child's vocalizations to increase appreciably in the school settings, where no parent was present to prompt or provide models to imitate.

Another study of parent teaching at home with generalization of child behaviors measured at school was reported by Wedel and Fowler (1984). Subjects in this study were higher-functioning than those in the Miller and Sloane (1976) study. Four mothers were taught to be home-tutors for their language-delayed children, aged 4 to 6 years. Parents were instructed to read and tape-record a story to their child four evenings a week. Books were preselected to ensure that they contained 10 to 15 examples of the words and letters that were the target behaviors for the child. Mothers were taught to stop at the end of each page, point to a target and ask the child to identify it. Correct responses were consequated with occasional praise, and for other responses mothers labeled the target and rehearsed it with the child. The parent trainer provided feedback on both the child's performance on school probes of the target and on the parents' performance as tutors, based on the tape recordings. Weekly generalization probes at school consisted of presentations of the targets, once from a storybook page and once on a flash card. New training sets were assigned after criterion was met on these probes.

Results indicated that parents spent an average of 8 or 9 minutes per day reading and discussing a story, except for one parent who averaged 20 minutes per day. The average number of trials presented ranged from 32 to 9. No generalization data for home-tutoring behavior by mothers were gathered. Generalization data on child targets at school showed rapid acquisition and maintenance of the trained sight words, which were not taught at school. One child learned 26 words over 14 weeks, and a second child learned 18 words over 14 weeks. One of the children whose targets were letter identifications learned 12 letters in 11 weeks, whereas the other child showed slower acquisition and was less cooperative during the school probes. Substantial gains on *Peabody Picture Vocabulary Test* (Dunn, 1965) scores were noted for the two children learning sight words, although whether these gains could be attributed directly to the home-reading program is not clear.

Clearly, a parent-child reading program can be an effective way to teach not only pre-reading and reading skills, but many kinds of oral language targets as well. Clinicians who have worked with parents may have some guidelines similar to those used by Wedel and Fowler to give parents who want suggestions for working with their children at home. If not, a set of specially selected children's books might be collected, with key vocabulary words, or semantic classes of words, or grammatical targets marked. Data collection sheets for language targets commonly taught to several children could be developed and given to parents. Assigning parents specific targets that are then *not* treated by the clinician, but only probed periodically, can show parents the effects of *their* teaching. The short periods required for book-reading may be attractive for parents who feel they do not have much time for working with their child.

One more idea that might be incorporated into a home-tutoring program is teaching the child a request for story reading. This would be an example of teaching a functional response, one that works to increase parent-child interaction and probably facilitates language learning by its very nature. Given cooperative parents, a functional request such as "Please read story" may serve as a mediator of generalized parent language-teaching strategies.

Conversational skills were targeted for treatment by the mother of a mentally retarded adolescent in a study by Arnold and co-workers (1977). Using a multiple-baseline design, the mother taught two classes of language behavior to the child: encouragements to talk (e.g., "I'll bet!" "Really!" "Yeah!") and on-topic questions. Teaching procedures included imitations of a model, verbal prompting, immediate feedback, and social reinforcement. Steps progressed from modeling and delayed imitation of encouragements to 4-minute conversations during which at least nine appropriate encouragements were produced. Similar steps were used during the teaching of questions. For parent training, the mother was seen for six 1-hour sessions in a clinic. After assessment data collection procedures were explained to her, the mother recorded seven 5-minute baseline interaction assessments in the home. Then explanations, discussions, observation of therapist-child interaction, and role-playing were used to train the mother to teach encouragements. Additional assessment data were gathered for analysis of both parent and child language behaviors. Frequency counts were made of the child's use of specific target skills and the mother's acknowledgments of those skills (e.g., "Terrific!" "You used one encouragement that time"). Training for teaching questions followed the same format as for teaching encouragements. Final tape-recorded assessment data were collected two months following the termination of parent training to determine generalization of both parent and child behaviors.

Results of this study indicated that the child's use of the language targets increased from baseline levels of 20 to 25 per cent median use during 5-minute conversational interactions to 42 to 44 per cent after treatment. At the two-month follow-up, median use was 35 per cent for encouragements, and 54 per cent for questions. Assessment data also indicated that the mother consistently acknowledged her daughter's correct responses and experienced no problems in systematically implementing the training steps. Unfortunately, no specific data on the mother's language behaviors during baseline or subsequent assessments were provided. However, the mother reported that she continued daily sessions after termination because she saw positive changes and enjoyed the interaction. Since the study was a multiple-baseline across behaviors, the encouragements target was used as a control during question teaching. The data indicated that use of encouragements decreased to baseline levels (28 per cent) when it was not being directly trained. This suggests that little maintenance was occurring. However, the two-month follow-up data were rather encouraging—especially for uses of questions.

This study by Arnold and colleagues provides some interesting strategies for designing and implementing language teaching programs with parent-child partners. The target behavior was well-chosen; encouragements and questions are appropriate pragmatic language targets. However, it would have been interesting to know whether the target behaviors generalized to conversational partners other than the mother who did not use acknowledgments as the mother did. Bringing a third person into the mother-child conversation would provide a measure of generalization of the conversational skills across persons. The use of parent-training in the clinic alleviates the need for a home-trainer, although this may not be the best method for training all parents.

The mother in the study by Arnold and co-workers (1977) continued her teaching strategies after the study ceased because she enjoyed the interaction. However, not all parents will find their teaching interactions to be intrinsically rewarding. Sometimes parents may require external rewards for working with their children. An interesting study that provided incentives for the parents to teach language targets was reported by Muir and Milan (1982). Just as children may need external reinforcers to motivate them to produce repetitions during therapy sessions, adults may also be more frequent and consistent in their teaching attempts if they are earning rewards. A number of commercial establishments provided coupons as lottery prizes for parents that were contingent on the accomplishments of their language-delayed children. Three single mothers and their 24- to 27-month-old children participated in the ABAB reversal design, which demonstrated effects of the parent reinforcement program. A series of eight early receptive language skills (e.g., responding to name, pointing to pictures) and five early expressive language skills (e.g., imitating vowels and consonants, naming objects) were operationally defined. For each behavior, the mother was taught an appropriate prompt and appropriate consequences for correct and incorrect responses.

An initial home visit established baseline child behaviors, and three behaviors not meeting criterion were assigned as tasks for the next home visit. Approximately once a week, the therapist tested each task for mastery three times in random order and provided modeling, feedback, and encouragement to enhance the mother's skills and participation. During the initial phase of the experiment, mothers were asked to provide instruction for the three tasks as often as possible throughout the week. Tasks mastered during this baseline-1 phase ranged from one to three. Then each mother was told that tickets for lottery prizes would be awarded for every task her child mastered, a maximum of three tickets for each visit. During the first lottery phase, children mastered 9, 9, and 5 tasks. Tasks mastered during the baseline-2 phase fell to 0 or 1, indicating that the lottery tickets were probably motivating the mothers and therefore their children were learning more tasks. A second lottery phase resulted in mastery of 10, 7, and 5 tasks for the three children. In all, the children mastered 643 per cent more tasks during the lottery conditions than during the baseline conditions (Muir and Milan, 1982).

Unfortunately, maintenance of parent teaching behaviors was not measured in this study, and if we assume that the baseline conditions were accurate measures of the effects of parent teaching when no lottery tickets were motivating them, then the results are disappointing. The mastery rates of the children were dramatically improved while the lottery phases were in effect, but not during the return to baseline. Thus, little maintenance or generalization of parent teaching behaviors across time must be presumed. Muir and Milan suggest that the results of their study argue against the assumption that improvement in their children's behavior is a powerful reinforcer for parents' instructional efforts. Rather, children's progress was maximized when progress-contingent reinforcement was earned by the mothers. Certainly, this conclusion does not apply to all parents, but the level of parents' motivation to work with the child needs to be considered on an individual basis. This issue is surely a controversial one and should be discussed among both professionals involved in early intervention efforts and parents themselves.

Recruiting Natural Communities of Reinforcement

Sometimes there are powerful reinforcing contingencies in some natural environments just waiting for appropriate language behavior to occur. For example, many people like to talk—give them a good listener and they can talk for hours. Some people like to converse with young children; they ask questions just to see what the child will say. Or perhaps they like to tease children, to see how big a story the child will believe before the leg-pulling is revealed. Consider for a moment the ready community of attention-givers that might be recruited for communicative interaction with language-handicapped children. If appropriate social language skills can be established in therapy and generalization strategies can be implemented to transfer them to other environments, these available reinforcers can serve to maintain appropriate language skills.

However, for various reasons, natural communities of reinforcement may have to be actively recruited rather then passively tapped. In one of the first studies of such active recruitment, delinquent girls were taught to prompt or cue the staff of an institution to evaluate and praise good work (Seymour and Stokes, 1976). A subsequent study applied a similar strategy to teach both normal preschoolers and slightly older deviant children to recruit praise for good work from classroom teachers (Stokes, Fowler, and Baer, 1978).

In the first of two experiments by Stokes and co-workers, normal preschoolers were taught to give cues (defined as statements inviting favorable comments or positive evaluation of work or behavior) after completing good work, by procedures such as instructions, role-playing, feedback, and praise. Good work was behaviorally defined (staying within lines, erasing errors, completing a page). Diverse cues (e.g., "Look how careful I've been" or "How is this work?") were taught to avoid mechanical, stereotyped responses. In addition, an optimal rate of two to four cues per 10-minute session was determined by consulting preschool teachers about what level of cues would be considered a nuisance. A multiple-baseline design across four subjects was used to determine the effects of training on cueing during generalization sessions. These sessions were conducted with two different teachers, who simply asked the children to work at their work sheets for the 10-minute sessions; these teachers were not told how to conduct the session.

Results of the first experiment indicated that spontaneous generalization from training sessions to generalization sessions occurred for only one child. Therefore, generalization programming was begun. The trainer, during the training session, instructed the child to work carefully in the generalization session, evaluate the work, and ask the teacher a few times about the quality of the work, but not too often. After the generalization session, children were asked if they had followed these instructions, and if they reported that they had done so, they earned a small toy. Since data were collected during the generalization sessions, accuracy of child-reports could be determined. When two of the four children reported inaccurately, they were gently confronted with "Are you sure?" or "I don't think you did," which resulted in accurate reports thereafter.

During training, the children's cues increased from a baseline of zero to frequencies of six to nine cues among the four children. After children were instructed to cue during the generalization sessions, cues in these sessions increased to frequencies of two to four cues during the 10-minute sessions. Thus, after generalization programming, the children generalized their cueing to natural academic interactions with teachers. As cues increased, so did teacher praise. This first experiment showed that children "were able to contact, recruit, and cultivate a dormant, but readily available natural community of increased reinforcement" (Stokes, Fowler, and Baer, 1978, p. 293).

In the second experiment, six-year-olds referred to a remedial summer class because of academic and behavior problems were taught to raise their hands and wait for the teacher to approach before cueing praise, and data for both appropriate (when the teacher was close) and inappropriate cueing were collected. Self-evaluation of work quality and diversity of cues were again emphasized in training the children. At the end of each training session, children were instructed to work and cue praise in the classroom setting the same as they had done in training. Children were also told to cue three times during the 20-minute work period in the classroom and to spread the cues across the work period. Later in the day, each child met with the trainer to report on his or her work and cueing and to earn a toy if he or she had carried out the instructions.

Results of this second experiment indicated that these children, like the normal preschoolers, learned to recruit praise at an appropriate frequency for good work. One child, observed seven months after completion of the experiment, cued his teacher in the special classroom three times in the 20-minute work period, indicating maintenance of the learned behavior. The inclusion of the hand-raise before cueing seemed to serve as a common (mediated) stimulus that facilitated cueing in the classroom setting, thus ensuring that some "spontaneous" generalization across settings occurred. One child showed a substantial rate of inappropriate cueing during baseline measures, and this rate decreased during the generalization programming. Thus, these delayed children generalized their cueing to a natural classroom setting, where more children competed for teacher attention and academic materials were diverse. In discussing the results of their study, Stokes and associates suggested some guidelines for applying this cueing strategy in various situations: consult with teachers about acceptable levels of cueing, discuss with the child the environmental tolerance for cueing, and ask the child to report on the cueing and the teacher's responses to it.

The child behaviors measured in the Stokes and co-workers (1978) study included both work skills and a specific language behavior, cueing teacher praise. The language behavior was successfully taught and with extra programming was also successfully generalized across settings and persons. It would be interesting to apply this recruitment of praise strategy to actual language behaviors rather than to work skills. For children who are working on language targets that require self-monitoring and self-correction, such as remembering to use a particular grammar target in obligatory contexts, to produce a certain polite form, or to stay on-topic during conversations, the cueing of praise or other reinforcement from listeners may be a good generalization strategy. The role of the clinician may be shifted from an initial strategy of direct intervention to teach the cueing language to a follow-up strategy of discussing the self-reports with the child or providing contingent delayed consequences for appropriate use of the cues, or both. Gradually, such delayed consequences should be faded as the child becomes an active agent of his or her own behavior change.

SELF-MONITORING AND MEDIATION

If we think for a moment about how we go about changing our own behavior, it becomes obvious that we use a form of self-monitoring. We set goals, break the goals down into smaller steps, keep track of our work toward that goal, and decide whether we need to change strategies or modify the goal based on some sort of evidence of progress or lack of it. A key element in changing our behavior is our ability to monitor it, i.e., to become aware of behaviors that help us reach the goal or hinder our progress toward the goal. Speech-language clinicians need to help clients learn self-monitoring skills and mediation strategies so they can apply them to maintaining therapy-taught language behaviors outside the treatment environment.

When self-monitoring skills are taught, part of the procedure is to use some recording method to keep track of opportunities to use the behavior and the accuracy with which the behavior was used. The presence of a recording device works as a mediator between the client and the behavior to be monitored. According to Holman and Baer (1979), mediation of transfer or generalization requires that a response be learned that will generate a stimulus in both training and nontraining environments. When that response is produced, a reinforcing stimulus occurs, thereby promoting generalization to nontreatment environments. If we can teach self-control or self-monitoring, then this procedure may become a strategy used by clients to promote their own behavior change over time, that is, to increase the durability of learned behavior.

Studies of self-monitoring of speech-language behaviors are hard to find. However, the procedure for teaching self-monitoring can be noted in a study of on-task behavior by Holman and Baer (1979). Three normal preschoolers and three older deviant children (learning deficits and behavior problems such as noncompliance, aggression, and hyperactivity) were taught self-monitoring skills to facilitate independent work habits, using a multiple-baseline design across subjects. Training was conducted in an experimental room, using a bracelet with movable beads to record completed pages of work. Treatment consisted of instructions to move a bead upon completing each page and to try to make it to a designated criterion bead. Praise was given for completing a page and remembering to move a bead; prompts to self-record were faded over the first five sessions. In the classroom (generalization setting), children were given the bracelet and the same instructions, but no praise or prompting. These generalization probes occurred later in the day, after the training session.

Results indicated that both normal and deviant children improved their on-task responding an average of 55 per cent over baseline levels. Effects, though variable, were observable almost immediately after treatment was applied. Levels of off-task behavior were reduced to about half their baseline levels for the normal subjects, but remained about the same for the deviant subjects.

Three of the original six subjects were available for follow-up probes of maintenance two months after treatment was terminated. Follow-up measures were collected twice weekly for three months, with three additional months of data collected on two of the subjects. A reversal design was used during follow-up measures to investigate the effects of withdrawing and returning the bracelet. One normal and one deviant subject showed durable benefits of training when the bracelet was present, although on-task behavior deteriorated when the bracelet was withdrawn. The third subject, a normal child, showed no maintenance. However, subsequent data indicated that this child's on-task behavior was under the control of his classroom peer, whose on-task behavior was mediated by the bracelet (Holman and Baer, 1979). Since low rates of teacher prompts and praise were observed for all phases of the study, increased on-task behavior was not due to teacher behaviors, but to children's responses to the bracelet.

In discussing the results of their study, Holman and Baer suggested that the transfer of work skills to the generalization setting was mediated primarily by the discriminative properties of the bracelet, which reminded the children to work, to complete a certain amount of work, to record progress, and to seek reinforcement from the teacher. When the bracelet was not present, these reminders did not occur, and on-task behavior decreased. Use of the bracelet-mediator tactic may provide a useful transition between therapy and classroom by facilitating generalization to a second setting without extensively altering that setting.

The mediator in the Stokes and associates (1978) study, in which children were taught to recruit praise for good work, was the hand-raise. Since hand-raising is a common occurrence in most classrooms, it served as a good prompt to say something that would elicit praise for good work from the teacher. When we think about how often normal children do this, at least when they are young, it seems a reasonable language behavior to teach language-handicapped children who can handle it.

Think now about applying this self-monitoring and mediating strategy to language behaviors. Language targets might be broken down into two categories. One category would include targets whose production frequency needs to be increased; i.e., they need to be used more often in appropriate circumstances. The other would include targets for which opportunities and attempts occur frequently, but for which the productions are often in error. Examples of the first kind of language target might be verbal requests for information, objects, or actions, appropriate comments within conversation, or appropriate application of semantic knowledge during academic tasks. Examples of the second might be grammatical errors such as omission of articles or auxiliaries or substitution of object-case for subject-case pronouns within sentences. For language targets that need to occur more frequently, some kind of reminder to produce the language behavior may be needed. Analysis of those circumstances in which the target would be appropriate may yield some appropriate stimuli for triggering the desired behavior.

Consider polite forms, such as "please" and "thank you." These are probably directly taught by parents to their normal children, although observational learning may also play a role. The stimuli that should trigger "please" might be the sight of some attractive object, the need for an action, or perhaps an internal feeling such as hunger or desire. If the child has learned that the probability that a request will be granted increases when "please" is added, then desirable, attractive stimuli may result in production of "please." The production of "thank you" may be a much simpler matter of learning a verbal routine that goes with "please." Take some common language targets or prelanguage targets and consider the occasions of their use. When are they likely to occur in the natural environment? What possible stimuli might elicit them? Once they are learned, what strategies can be used to ensure that they will occur spontaneously in the natural environments?

Instead of trying to figure out a single "controlling stimulus," remember that learning does not occur in a vacuum. In natural environments especially, behaviors often *only* occur in the right context. Language behaviors, in particular, are likely to occur only in the right context. In the therapy room we can often arrange those "right contexts" by controlling the visual and verbal stimuli, the person, the setting, and the reinforcement or consequences. However, those factors or combinations of factors may never be found in natural environments, let alone be under the clinician's control! The best we can hope for may be to allow a number of possible factors to vary and see if the language behavior will occur under a wide variety of conditions. Of course, then, there is the chance that it will occur when it *should not* occur. We want a robust language behavior that will be used whenever appropriate circumstances occur, but not an indiscriminant one that will occur in inappropriate circumstances. Achieving generalization of language behaviors is a tricky business.

CONCLUSIONS

The aim of this book has been to help practicing speech-language clinicians anticipate and prepare for problems in generalization of language target behaviors. If we are aware that the targets we choose to work on in our therapy sessions may be displayed only in therapy situations, we can plan ahead to avoid some problems and implement procedures to increase generalization when it is limited. It may be helpful to ask ourselves some questions about the language targets we are considering for each client (or the ones we have already chosen) before we begin therapy. The questions listed in Table 8–3 are suggested as aids in designing intervention programs that will include generalization strategies early in the treatment process. They may be viewed as a summary of major principles for implementing generalization strategies.

It may not be easy, however, to implement some of the various strategies presented in this book. Often the sites in which therapy is administered are not amenable to change. Perhaps no funds are available for altering the therapy setting, or co-workers may object to your carrying out therapy in a variety of places. Parents or ward aids may not be interested in providing extra opportunities for practicing the language target behavior or may not be willing to (or remember to) respond in necessary ways to a client's correct or incorrect attempts at producing the language target. Perhaps your attempts to get your clients to self-monitor will result in numerous lost counters or notebooks and all kinds of excuses about why your recommendations were not remembered or carried out.

Nevertheless, attempts to implement some generalization strategies must be made if treatment efforts are to result in generalized and maintained responses. Perhaps some changes can be made in data collection procedures to include several measures of generalization and response maintenance. A system for checking generalization and maintenance might be worked out with other speech-language clinicians in your work setting or neighboring settings. Supervisors, psychologists, social workers, or other special educators may be willing to help in implementing some generalization strategies, depending on the work setting. Make it a team effort, so that both successes and failures can be shared. Revise strategies that do not seem to be effective after brainstorming with colleagues about possible reasons for failure.

As clinicians begin to alter language intervention planning so that generalization strategies are implemented earlier in the process, the "clinician's dilemma" should decrease. The hours of treatment, whether spent in one-to-one therapy during the establishment phase, in data collection in nontreatment settings with nontreatment persons, or in parent training efforts during a generalization phase, should pay off with appropriately generalized language behaviors produced in a variety of natural environments. By anticipating generalization problems and planning early to overcome them, we can provide intervention that will

Table 8–3. Questions to Ask Before Beginning Treatment

1. Is the target behavior one that will be functional and frequently usable in several nontreatment (natural) environments?
2. What kinds of antecedent events already occur in natural environments that set the occasion for production of the language target under consideration? Could these naturally occurring antecedent events be brought into your treatment situaion?
3. How often do the antecedent events occur in a typical day or week? Could that frequency be increased so that there are more opportunities to practice the language target behavior?
4. What kinds of consequent events already occur in natural environments when the language target is produced? If the target under consideration is never produced, what behaviors is the client substituting for it? What consequent events follow these substitute behaviors? Could they be changed?
5. What kinds of consequent events already occur in natural environments when an error in the language target occurs? When the target is grammatically correct production of sentences, what are the consequent events following grammatical errors within natural environments? Is the message content attended to, with grammatical form ignored? Do listeners expand the sentence or provide a correct model?
6. What are several possible settings in which measures of generalization of targets under consideration might be easily gathered? Could these settings be turned into extensions of treatment if generalization does not occur?
7. Who are several persons with whom measures of generalization of targets might easily be gathered? Could these persons be incorporated into treatment programs if generalization does not occur? Can these persons be recruited to provide prompts and opportunities for display of language targets? Can they be taught to deliver appropriate consequent events for correct and incorrect productions of the target?

achieve a major goal, "... to teach a repertoire of communication skills that will be used outside training, with persons who are not trainers, to describe objects and events that are usually physically different from, but conceptually similar to, those described in training" (Rogers-Warren and Warren, 1981, p. 390).

References

Arnold, S., Sturgis, E., and Forehand, R. (1977). Training a parent to teach communication skills: A case study. *Behavior Modification, 1*, 259–276.

Baer, D. (1981). *How to plan for generalization*. Lawrence, KS: H and H Enterprises.

Bandura, A., and Harris, M. (1966). Modification of syntactic style. *Journal of Experimental Child Psychology, 4*, 341–352.

Bates, E., Camaioni, L., and Volterra, V. (1975). The acquisition of performatives prior to speech. *Merrill-Palmer Quarterly, 21*, 205–216.

Bayley, N. (1969). *Bayley Scales of Infant Development: Birth to two years.* New York: Psychological Corporation.

Bennett, C., and Ling, D. (1972). Teaching a complex verbal response to a hearing-impaired girl. *Journal of Applied Behavior Analysis, 5*, 321–327.

Brinker, R., and Bricker, D. (1979). Teaching a first language: building complex structures from simpler components. In J. Mittler and P. Hogg (Eds.), *Advances in mental handicap research* (pp. 197–223). New York: Wiley.

Brown, R. (1973). *A first language: The early stages.* Cambridge, MA: Harvard University Press.

Bucher, B., and Keller, M. (1981). Transfer to productive labeling after training in comprehension: Effects of three training variables. *Analysis and Intervention in Developmental Disabilities, 1*, 315–331.

Bzoch, K., and League, R. (1971). *The Receptive-Expressive Emergent Language Scale for the measurement of language skills in infancy.* Gainesville, FL: Tree of Life Press.

Campbell, C., and Stremel-Campbell, K. (1982). Programming "loose training" as a strategy to facilitate language generalization. *Journal of Applied Behavior Analysis, 15*, 295–301.

Carr, E. (1980). Generalization of treatment effects following educational intervention with autistic children and youth. In B. Wilcox and A. Thompson (Eds.), *Critical issues in educating autistic children and youth* (pp. 118–134). Washington, D.C.: U. S. Department of Education.

Carr, E., and Kologinsky, E. (1983). Acquisition of sign language by autistic children II: Spontaneity and generalization effects. *Journal of Applied Behavior Analysis, 16*, 297–314.

Carr, E., Newsom, C., and Binkoff, J. (1980). Escape as a factor in the aggressive behavior of two retarded children. *Journal of Applied Behavior Analysis, 13*, 113–129.

Carroll, W., Rosenthal, T., and Brysh, C. (1972). Social transmission of grammatical parameters. *Journal of Educational Psychology, 63*, 589–578.

Clark, H., and Sherman, J. (1975). Teaching generative use of sentence answers to three forms of questions. *Journal of Applied Behavior Analysis, 8*, 321–330.

Connell, P. (1982). On training language rules. *Language, Speech, and Hearing Services in Schools, 13*, 231–240.
Connell, P., and McReynolds, L. (1981). An experimental analysis of children's generalization during lexical learning: Comprehension or production. *Applied Psycholinguistics, 2*, 309–332.
Courtright, J., and Courtright, I. (1976). Imitative modeling as theoretical base for instructing language-disordered children. *Journal of Speech and Hearing Research, 19*, 655–663.
Courtright, J., and Courtright, I. (1979). Imitative modeling as a language intervention strategy: The effects of two mediating variables. *Journal of Speech and Hearing Research, 22*, 389–402.
Costello, J. (1983). Generalization across settings. In J. Miller, D. Yoder, and R. Schiefelbusch (Eds.), *Contemporary issues in language intervention* (ASHA Reports, No. 12) (pp. 275–297). Rockville, MD: American Speech and Hearing Association.
Crabtree, M. (1963). *Houston test for language development*. Chicago: Stoelting.
Cromer, C., and Ault, R. (1979). Generalization in the receptive and productive language of preschool children. *Journal of Educational Research, 73*, 31–36.
Crystal, D. (1983). Psycholinguistics. *Folia Phoniatrica, 35*, 1–12.
Culatta, B., and Horn, D. (1982). A program for achieving generalization of grammatical rules to spontaneous discourse. *Journal of Speech and Hearing Disorders, 47*, 174–180.
Culatta, B., and Page, J. (1982). Strategies for achieving generalization of grammatical constructions. *Communicative Disorders, 7*, 31–44.
Cuvo, A., and Riva, M. (1980). Generalization and transfer between comprehension and production: A comparison of retarded and nonretarded persons. *Journal of Applied Behavior Analysis, 13*, 315–332.
Drabman, R., Hammer, D., and Rosenbaum, M. (1979). Assessing generalization in behavior modification with children: The generalization map. *Behavioral Assessment, 1*, 203–219.
Duker, P., and Morsink, H. (1984). Acquisition and cross-setting generalization of manual signs with severely retarded individuals. *Journal of Applied Behavior Analysis, 17*, 93–104.
Egel, A. (1981). Programming the generalization and maintenance of treatment gains. In R. Koegel, A. Rincover, and A. Egel (Eds.), *Educating and understanding autistic children* (pp. 281–299). Houston, TX: College-Hill Press.
Faw, G., Reid, D., Schepis, M., Fitzgerald, J., and Welty, P. (1981). Involving institutional staff in the development and maintenance of sign language skills with profoundly retarded persons. *Journal of Applied Behavior Analysis, 14*, 411–423.
Forehand, R., Atkeson, B. (1977). Generality of treatment effects with parents as therapists: A review of assessment and implementation procedures. *Behavior Therapy, 8*, 575–593.
Foxx, R., McMorrow, M., and Mennemeier, M. (1984). Teaching social/vocational skills to retarded adults with a modified table game: An analysis of generalization. *Journal of Applied Behavior Analysis, 17*, 343–352.
Foxx, R., McMorrow, M., and Schloss, C. (1983). Stacking the deck: Teaching social skills to retarded adults with a modified table game. *Journal of Applied Behavior Analysis, 16*, 157–170.
Fygetakis, L., and Gray, B. (1970). Programmed conditioning of linguistic competence. *Behaviour Research and Therapy, 8*, 153–163.

Fygetakis, L., and Ingram, D. (1973). Language rehabilitation and programmed conditioning: A case study. *Journal of Learning Disabilities, 6,* 60–64.

Gajar, A., Schloss, P., Schloss, C., and Thompson, C. (1984). Effects of feedback and self-monitoring on head trauma youths' conversation skills. *Journal of Applied Behavior Analysis, 17,* 353–358.

Garcia, E. (1974). The training and generalization of a conversational speech form in nonverbal retardates. *Journal of Applied Behavior Analysis, 7,* 137–149.

Garcia, E., Bullet, J., and Rust, F. (1977). An experimental analysis of language training generalization across classroom and home. *Behavior Modification, 1,* 531–549.

Garcia, E., and DeHaven, E. (1974). Use of operant techniques in the establishment and generalization of language: A review and analysis. *American Journal of Mental Deficiency,* 79, 169–178.

Garcia, E., Guess, D., and Byrnes, J. (1973). Development of syntax in a retarded girl using procedures of imitation, reinforcement, and modeling. *Journal of Applied Behavior Analysis, 6,* 299–310.

Gaylord-Ross, R., Harring, T., Breen, C., and Pitts-Conway, V. (1984). The training and generalization of social interaction skills with autistic youth. *Journal of Applied Behavior Analysis, 17,* 229–247.

Gray, B., and Fygetakis, L. (1968). The development of language as a function of programmed conditioning. *Behaviour Research and Therapy, 6,* 455–460.

Gray, B., and Ryan, B. (1973). *A language program for the nonlanguage child.* Champaign, IL: Research Press.

Guess, D. (1969). A functional analysis of receptive language and productive speech: Acquisition of the plural morpheme. *Journal of Applied Behavior Analysis, 2,* 55–64.

Guess, D., and Baer, D. (1973). An analysis of individual differences in generalization between receptive and productive language in retarded children. *Journal of Applied Behavior Analysis, 6,* 311–329.

Guess, D., Keough, W., and Sailor, D. (1978). Generalization of speech and language behavior: Measurement and training tactics. In R. Schiefelbusch (Ed.), *Bases of language intervention* (pp. 374–395). Baltimore: University Park Press.

Guess, D., Sailor, W., and Baer, D. (1976–1978). *Functional speech and language training for the severely handicapped* (Parts 1–4). Lawrence, KS: H and H Enterprises.

Guess, D., Sailor, W., Rutherford, G., and Baer, D. (1968). An experimental analysis of linguistic development: the productive use of the plural morpheme. *Journal of Applied Behavior Analysis, 1,* 297–306.

Handleman, J. (1979). Generalization by autistic-type children of verbal responses across settings. *Journal of Applied Behavior Analysis, 12,* 273–282.

Handleman, J. (1981). Transfer of verbal responses across instructional settings by autistic-type children. *Journal of Speech and Hearing Disorders, 46,* 69–76.

Handleman, J., Powers, M., and Harris, S. (1984). Teaching of labels: An analysis of concrete and pictorial representations. *American Journal of Mental Deficiency, 88,* 625–629.

Harris, D., Lippert, J., Yoder, D., and Vanderheiden, G. (1979). Blissymbolics: An augmentative symbol communication system for nonvocal severely hand-

icapped children. In R. York and E. Edgar (Eds.), *Teaching the severely handicapped*. Columbus, OH: Special Press.
Hart, B. (1980). Pragmatics and language development. In B. Lahey and A. Kazdin (Eds.), *Advances in clinical child psychology,* Vol. 3 (pp. 383–427). New York: Plenum Press.
Hart, B. (1981). Pragmatics: How language is used. *Analysis and Intervention in Developmental Disabilities, 1*, 299–313.
Hart, B., and Risley, T. (1968). Establishing use of descriptive adjectives in the spontaneous speech of disadvantaged preschool children. *Journal of Applied Behavior Analysis, 1,* 109–120.
Hart, B., and Risley, T. (1974). The use of preschool materials for modifying the language of disadvantaged children. *Journal of Applied Behavior Analysis, 7,* 243–256.
Hart, B., and Risley, T. (1975). Incidental teaching of language in the preschool. *Journal of Applied Behavior Analysis, 8*, 411–420.
Hart, B., and Risley, T. (1980). In vivo language intervention: Unanticipated general effects. *Journal of Applied Behavior Analysis, 13*, 407–432.
Hart, B., and Risley, T. (1982). *How to use incidental teaching for elaborating language*. Lawrence, KS: H and H Enterprises.
Hart, B., and Rogers-Warren, A. (1978). A milieu approach to teaching language. In R. Schiefelbusch (Ed.), *Language intervention strategies* (pp. 193–235). Baltimore: University Park Press.
Haynes, W., and Haynes, M. (1980). A comparison of nonimitative modeling and mimicry procedures for training the singular copula in black preschool children. *Journal of Communication Disorders, 13*, 277–288.
Hegde, M. N. (1985). *Treatment principles and procedures in communicative disorders*. San Diego: College-Hill Press.
Hegde, M. (1980). An experimental-clinical analysis of grammatical and behavioral distinctions between verbal auxiliary and copula. *Journal of Speech and Hearing Research, 23*, 864–877.
Hegde, M., and Gierut, J. (1979). The operant training and generalization of pronouns and a verb form in a language-delayed child. *Journal of Communication Disorders, 12*, 23–34.
Hegde, M., and McConn, J. (1981). Language training: Some factors affecting generalization to an occupational setting. *Journal of Speech and Hearing Disorders, 46*, 353–358.
Hegde, M., Noll, M., and Pecora, R. (1979). A study of some factors affecting generalization of language training. *Journal of Speech and Hearing Disorders, 44*, 301–320.
Hendrickson, J., Strain, P., Tremblay, A., and Shores, R. (1982). Interactions of behaviorally handicapped children: Functional effects of peer social initiations. *Behavior Modification, 6*, 323–353.
Holdgrafer, G., and McReynolds, L. (1975, Autumn). An experimental analysis of comprehension and production in children's acquisition of morphological rules. *Human Communication,* p. 61.
Holman, J., and Baer, D. (1979). Facilitating generalization of on-task behavior through self-monitoring of academic tasks. *Journal of Autism and Developmental Disorders, 9*, 429–446.
Hughes, D. (1982). *The effects of two syntax treatment programs on rate of target generalization to spontaneous language*. Unpublished doctoral dissertation, University of Washington.

Johnston, J. (1982). Generalization: The nature of change. In *Proceedings of the third Wisconsin symposium on research in child language disorders,* Madison, WI.

Karlan, G., Brenn-White, B., Lentz, A., Hodur, P., Egger, D., and Frankoff, D. (1982). Establishing generalized, productive verb-noun phrase usage in a manual language system with moderately handicapped children. *Journal of Speech and Hearing Disorders, 47,* 31–42.

Kazdin, A. (1977). *The token economy: A review and evaluation.* New York: Plenum Press.

Kazdin, A. (1980). *Behavior modification in applied settings* (2nd ed.). Homewood, IL: Dorsey Press.

Kazdin, A., and Esveldt-Dawson, K. (1981). *How to maintain behavior.* Lawrence, KS: H and H Enterprises.

Keilitz, I., Tucker, D., and Horner, R. (1973). Increasing mentally retarded adolescents' verbalizations about current events. *Journal of Applied Behavior Analysis, 6,* 621–630.

Keller, M., and Bucher, B. (1979). Transfer between receptive and productive language in developmentally disabled children. *Journal of Applied Behavior Analysis, 12,* 311.

Koegel, R., and Rincover, A. (1974). Treatment of psychotic children in a classroom environment: I. Learning in a large group. *Journal of Applied Behavior Analysis, 7,* 45–59.

Koegel, R., and Rincover, A. (1977). Research on the difference between generalization and maintenance in extra-therapy responding. *Journal of Applied Behavior Analysis, 10,* 1–12.

Koegel, R., Schreibman, L., Bitten, K., Burke, J., and O'Neil, R. (1981). A comparison of parent training to direct child treatment. In R. Koegel, A. Rincover, and A. Egel (Eds.). *Educating and understanding autistic children* (pp. 260–279). Houston, TX: College-Hill Press.

Kyne, J. (1980). The evolving parent-professional relationship. In B. Wilcox and A. Thompson (Eds.). *Critical issues in educating autistic children and youth* (pp. 234–240). Washington, DC: U. S. Department of Education.

Larson, V. (1983). Presentation on Adolescent Language at Annual Clinician's Workshop, Central Michigan University, Mt. Pleasant.

Leonard, L. (1975). Modeling as a clinical procedure in language training. *Language, Speech, and Hearing Services in Schools, 6,* 72–85.

Leonard, L. (1981). Facilitating linguistic skills in children with specific language impairment. *Applied Psycholinguistics, 2,* 89–118.

Leonard, L., Cole, B., and Steckol, K. (1979). Lexical usage of retarded children: An examination of informativeness. *American Journal of Mental Deficiency, 84,* 49–54.

Lovaas, O. (1981). *Teaching developmentally disabled children: The me book.* Baltimore: University Park Press.

Lovaas, O., Koegel, R., Simmons, J., and Stevens-Long, J. (1973). Some generalization and follow-up measures on autistic children in behavior therapy. *Journal of Applied Behavior Analysis, 6,* 131–166.

Lutzker, L., and Sherman, J. (1974). Producing generative sentence usage by imitation and reinforcement procedures. *Journal of Applied Behavior Analysis, 7,* 447–460.

Mahoney, G., and Snow, K. (1983). The relationship of sensorimotor functioning to children's response to early language training. *Mental Retardation,*

21, 248–254.

MacDonald, J. D., and Nickols, M. (1978). *Environmental language inventory.* Columbus, OH: Charles E. Merrill.

Marholin, D., II, and Siegel, L. (1978). Beyond the law of effect: Programming for the maintenance of behavioral change. In D. Marholin II (Ed.), *Child behavior therapy* (pp. 397–415). New York: Gardner Press.

Marholin, D., II, Siegel, L., and Phillips, D. (1976). Treatment and transfer: A search for empirical procedures. In M. Hersen, R. Eisler, and P. Miller (Eds.), *Progress in behavior modification* (pp. 293–342). New York: Academic Press.

Martin, J. (1975). Generalizing the use of descriptive adjectives through modeling. *Journal of Applied Behavior Analysis, 8*, 203–209.

Matson, J., and Earnhart, T. (1981). Programming treatment effects to the natural environment: A procedure for training institutionalized retarded adults. *Behavior Modification, 5*, 27–37.

McCormick, L., and Schiefelbusch, R. (1984). *Early language intervention: An introduction*. Columbus, OH: Charles E. Merrill.

McCuller, W., and Salzberg, C. (1984). Generalized action-object verbal instruction-following by profoundly mentally retarded adults. *American Journal of Mental Deficiency, 88*, 442–445.

McGee, G., Krantz, P., Mason, D., and McClannahan, L. (1983). A modified incidental-teaching procedure for autistic youth: Acquisition and generalization of receptive object labels. *Journal of Applied Behavior Analysis, 16*, 329–338.

McLean, J., Snyder-McLean, L., and Sack, S. (1981). *A transactional approach to early language: A mediated training program for pre-service and inservice professionals.* Columbus, OH: Charles E. Merrill.

McReynolds, L., and Engmann, D. (1974). An experimental analysis of the relationship of subject and object noun phrases. In L. McReynolds (Ed.), *Developing systematic procedures for training children's language* (ASHA Monographs, No. 18) (pp. 30–46). Rockville, MD: American Speech and Hearing Association.

McReynolds, L., and Kearns, K. (1983). *Single-subject experimental designs in communicative disorders*. Baltimore: University Park Press.

Miller, M., Cuvo, A., and Borakove, L. (1977). Teaching naming of coin values: Comprehension before production vs. production alone. *Journal of Applied Behavior Analysis, 10*, 135.

Miller, S., and Sloane, H. (1976). The generalization effects of parent training across stimulus settings. *Journal of Applied Behavior Analysis, 9*, 355–370.

Mowrer, D. E. (1977). *Methods of modifying speech behaviors*. Columbus, OH: Charles E. Merrill.

Muir, K., and Milan, M. (1982). Parent reinforcement for child achievement: The use of a lottery to maximize parent training effects. *Journal of Applied Behavior Analysis, 15*, 455–460.

Mulac, A., and Tomlinson, C. (1977). Generalization of an operant remediation program for syntax with language-delayed children. *Journal of Communication Disorders*, 10, 231–243.

Oliver, P., and Scott, T. (1981). Group versus individual training in establishing generalization of language skills with severely handicapped individuals. *Mental Retardation, 19*, 285–289.

Olswang, L., Bain, B., Dunn, C., and Cooper, J. (1983). The effects of stimulus variation on lexical learning. *Journal of Speech and Hearing Disorders, 48*, 192–201.

Olswang, L., Kriegsmann, E., and Mastergeorge, A. (1982). Facilitating functional requesting in pragmatically impaired children. *Language, Speech, and Hearing Services in Schools, 13*, 202–222.

Paluszek, S., and Feintuch, F. (1979). Comparing imitation and comprehension training in two language-impaired children. *Working Papers in Experimental Speech-Language Pathology and Audiology, 8*, 72–91.

Prelock, P., and Panagos, J. (1980). Mimicry versus imitative modeling: Facilitating sentence production in the speech of the retarded. *Journal of Psycholinguistic Research, 9*, 565–578.

Prior, M., Minnes, P., Coyne, T., Golding, B., Hendy, J., and McGillivary, J. (1979). Verbal interactions between staff and residents in an institution for the young mentally retarded. *Mental Retardation, 17*, 65–69.

Rees, N. (1978). Pragmatics of language. In R. Schiefelbusch (Ed.), *Bases of language intervention* (pp. 191–268). Baltimore: University Park Press.

Rincover, A., and Koegel, R. (1975). Setting generality and stimulus control in autistic children. *Journal of Applied Behavior Analysis, 8*, 235–246.

Rogers-Warren, A., and Warren, S. (1980). Mands for verbalization: Facilitating the generalization of newly trained language in children. *Behavior Modification, 4*, 230–245.

Rogers-Warren, A., and Warren, S. (1981). Form and function in language learning and generalization. *Analysis and Intervention in Developmental Disabilities, 1*, 389–404.

Romski, M., and Ruder, K. (1984). Effects of speech and speech-and-sign instruction on oral language learning and generalization of action + object combinations by Down's syndrome children. *Journal of Speech and Hearing Disorders, 49*, 293–302.

Rubin, B., and Stolz, S. (1974). Generalization of self-referent speech established in a retarded adolescent by operant procedures. *Behavior Therapy, 5*, 93–106.

Ruder, K., Bunce, B., and Ruder, C. (1984). Language intervention in a preschool/classroom setting. In L. McCormick and R. Schiefelbusch, (Eds.), *Early language intervention: An introduction* (pp. 267–297). Columbus, OH: Charles E. Merrill.

Ruder, K., Smith, M., and Hermann, P. (1974). Effect of verbal imitation and comprehension on verbal production of lexical items. In L. McReynolds (Ed.), *Developing systematic procedures for training children's language* (ASHA Monographs, No. 18) Rockville, MD: American Speech and Hearing Association.

Ruder, K., Hermann, P., and Schiefelbusch, R. (1977). Effects of verbal imitation and comprehension training on verbal production. *Journal of Psycholinguistic Research, 6*, 59–72.

Rychtarik, R., and Bornstein, P. (1979). Training conversational skills in mentally retarded adults: A multiple baseline analysis. *Mental Retardation, 17*, 289–293.

Sailor, W. (1971). Reinforcement and generalization of productive plural allomorphs in two retarded children. *Journal of Applied Behavior Analysis, 4*, 305–310.

Schreibman, L., and Carr, E. (1978). Elimination of echolalic responding to questions through the training of a generalized verbal response. *Journal of Applied Behavior Analysis, 11*, 453–463.

Schumaker, J., and Sherman, J. (1970). Training generative verb usage by imitation and reinforcement procedures. *Journal of Applied Behavior Analysis, 3*, 273–287.

Senatore, V., Matson, J., and Kazdin, A. (1982). A comparison of behavioral methods to train social skills to mentally retarded adults. *Behavior Therapy, 13*, 313–324.

Seymour, F., and Stokes, T. (1976). Self-recording in training girls to increase work and evoke staff praise in an institution for offenders. *Journal of Applied Behavior Analysis, 9*, 41–54.

Skinner, B. F. (1953). *Science and human behavior.* New York: The Free Press.

Sosne, J., Handleman, J., and Harris, S. (1979). Teaching spontaneous-functional speech to autistic-type children. *Mental Retardation, 17*, 241–245.

Spradlin, J., and Siegel, G. (1982). Language training in natural and clinical environments. *Journal of Speech and Hearing Disorders, 47*, 2–6.

Stevens-Long, J., and Rasmussen, M. (1974). The acquisition of simple and compound sentence structure in an autistic child. *Journal of Applied Behavior Analysis, 7*, 473–479.

Stevens-Long, J., Schwarz, R., and Bliss, D. (1976). The acquisition and generalization of compound sentence structure in an autistic child. *Behavior Therapy, 7*, 397–404.

Stokes, T., and Baer, D. (1977). An implicit technology of generalization. *Journal of Applied Behavior Analysis, 10*, 349–367.

Stokes, T., Fowler, S., and Baer, D. (1978). Training preschool children to recruit natural communities of reinforcement. *Journal of Applied Behavior Analysis, 11*, 285–303.

Strain, P. (1977). Effects of peer social initiations on withdrawn preschool children: Some training and generalization effects. *Journal of Abnormal Child Psychology, 5*, 445–455.

Strain, P. (1980). Social behavior programming with severely handicapped and autistic children. In B. Wilcox and A. Thompson (Eds.), *Critical issues in educating autistic children and youth* (pp. 179–206). Washington, DC: U. S. Department of Education.

Strain, P., Kerr, M., and Ragland, E. (1979). Effects of peer-mediated social initiations and prompting/reinforcement procedures on the social behavior of autistic children. *Journal of Autism and Developmental Disorders, 9*, 41–54.

Strain, P., Shores, R., and Timm, M. (1977). Effects of peer initiations on the social behavior of withdrawn preschool children. *Journal of Applied Behavior Analysis, 10*, 289–298.

Stremel, K., and Waryas, C. (1974). A behavioral-psycholinguistic approach to language training. In L. McReynolds (Ed.), *Developing systematic procedures for training children's language* (pp. 96–130). Rockville, MD: ASHA Monographs No. 18.

Striefel, S., Wetherby, B., and Karlan, G. (1976). Establishing generative verb-noun instruction-following behavior in retarded children. *Journal of Experimental Child Psychology*, 22, 247–260.

Striefel, S., Wetherby, B., and Karlan, G. (1978). Developing generalized instruction-following behavior in the severely retarded. In C. E. Meyers (Ed.), *Quality of life in profoundly and severely retarded persons: Research foundation for improvement*. (American Association on Mental Deficiency Monograph Series No. 3.) Washington, DC: American Association on Mental Deficiency.

Thomson, N., Fraser, D., and McDougall, A. (1974). The reinstatement of speech in near-mute chronic schizophrenics by instructions, imitative prompts, and reinforcement. *Journal of Behavior Therapy and Experimental Psychiatry, 5*, 77–80.

Tremblay, A., Strain, P., Hendrickson, J., and Shores, R. (1981). Social interactions of normal preschool children: Using normative data for subject and target behavior selection. *Behavior Modification, 5*, 237–253.

Twardosz, A., and Baer, D. (1973). Training two severely retarded adolescents to ask questions. *Journal of Applied Behavior Analysis, 6*, 655–661.

Tyack, D., and Gottsleben, R. (1974). *Language sampling, analysis, and training*. Palo Alto, CA: Consulting Psychologists Press.

Uzgiris, I. C., and Hunt, J. McV. (1975). *Assessment in infancy: Ordinal scales of psychological development*. Urbana, IL: University of Illinois Press.

Wahler, R., Berland, R., and Coe, T. (1979). Generalization processes in child behavior change. In B. Lahey and A. Kazdin (Eds.), *Advances in clinical child psychology* (Vol. 2) (pp. 35–69). New York: Plenum Press.

Warren, S., Baxter, D., Anderson, S., Marshall, A., and Baer, D. (1981). Generalization of question-asking by severely retarded individuals. *TASH Journal, 6*, 15–22.

Warren, S., McQuarter, R., and Rogers-Warren, A. (1984). The effects of mands and models on the speech of unresponsive language-delayed preschool children. *Journal of Speech and Hearing Disorders, 49*, 34–51.

Warren, S., and Rogers-Warren, A. (1983a). A longitudinal analysis of language generalization among adolescents with severely handicapping conditions. *TASH Journal, 8*, 18–31.

Warren, S., and Rogers-Warren, A. (1983b). Because no one asked...: Setting variables effecting the generalization of trained vocabulary within a residential institution. In K. T. Kernan, M. J. Begab, and R. B. Edgerton (Eds.), *Environments and behavior: The adaptation of mentally retarded persons*. Baltimore: University Park Press.

Warren, S., Rogers-Warren, A., Baer, D., and Guess, D. (1980). Assessment and facilitation of language generalization. In W. Sailor, B. Wilcox, and L. Brown (Eds.), *Methods of instruction for severely handicapped students* (pp. 227–258). Baltimore: Brookes.

Warren, S., Rogers-Warren, A., and Buchanan, B. (1981, April). *A longitudinal analysis of comprehensive language training: Generalization to the real world*. Paper presented at the biannual meeting of the Society for Research in Child Development, Boston.

Wedel, J., and Fowler, S. (1984). "Read me a story, mom": A home-tutoring program to teach prereading skills to language-delayed children. *Behavior Modification, 8*, 245–266.

Welch, S. (1981). Teaching generative grammar to mentally retarded children: A review and analysis of a decade of behavioral research. *Mental Retardation, 19*, 277–284.

Welch, S., and Pear, J. (1980). Generalization of naming responses to objects in the natural environment as a function of training stimulus modality with retarded children. *Journal of Applied Behavior Analysis, 13*, 629–643.

Wheeler, A., and Sulzer, B. (1970). Operant training and generalization of a verbal response form in a speech-deficient child. *Journal of Applied Behavior Analysis, 3*, 139–147.

Wilcox, M., and Leonard, L. (1978). Experimental acquisition of *wh-* questions in language-disordered children. *Journal of Speech and Hearing Research, 21*, 220–239.

Zwitman, D., and Sonderman, J. (1979). A syntax program designed to present base linguistic structures to language-disordered children. *Journal of Communication Disorders, 12*, 323–355.

Author Index

T

U

V

W

Y

Z

Subject Index

Page numbers in italics refer to tables.

D

E

F

M

N

O

S

T

U

V

W